D1191036

NONOPERATIVE ASPECTS

OF

PEDIATRIC SURGERY

NONOPERATIVE ASPECTS

OF

PEDIATRIC SURGERY

With

Special Emphasis on Surgical Neonatology

By

RICHARD S. OWINGS, B.S., M.D., F.A.C.S., F.A.A.P.

Assistant Professor of Pediatrics
Instructor in Surgery
Medical College of Georgia
Augusta, Georgia

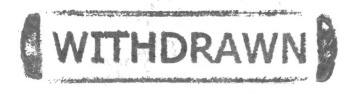
WITHDRAWN

WARREN H. GREEN, INC.

St. Louis, Missouri, U.S.A.

Published by

WARREN H. GREEN, INC.
10 South Brentwood Boulevard
Saint Louis, Missouri, U. S. A.

All rights reserved

© 1973 by WARREN H. GREEN, INC.

Library of Congress Catalog Card Number 72-176176

Printed in the United States of America

RD
137
.O98

DEDICATION

I would like to dedicate this book to all those physicians, nurses, medical students, interns, residents, parents and patients who have played such a vital role in allowing me to accumulate the information presented here.

I would also like to re-state the dedication made by the late Dr. Willis Potts in his *The Surgeon and The Child:*

> "to the infant who has the great misfortune of being born with a serious deformity. All life is before him, and what is done during the first few days may decide whether life will be a joy or a burden. If this infant could speak, it would beg imploringly of the surgeon, 'please exercise the greatest gentleness with my miniature tissues and try to correct the deformity at the first operation. Give me blood and the proper amount of fluid and electrolytes; add plenty of oxygen to the anesthesia, and I will show you that I can tolerate a terrific amount of surgery. You will be surprised at the speed of my recovery, and I shall always be grateful to you.' "

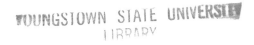
YOUNGSTOWN STATE UNIVERSITY
LIBRARY

323779

INTRODUCTION

To be honest with oneself, it is necessary to acknowledge that all the bits and pieces of knowledge one possesses has come from others. No effort will be made to disguise the origin of certain information in this book and there will be frequent direct quotes or paraphrasing, particularly when the author feels that no improvement is indicated in a particular method of presentation.

Subjects will not be divided into the divisions of the human body but the material for discussion will be limited to those non-operative problems and/or topics in pediatric surgery which are most important in the opinion of the author.

The following is from the Foreword to *The Essentials of Paediatric Surgery,* by the late Sir Denis Browne, FRCS:

"One of the rapidly developing sections of surgery . . . (is that section) . . . concentrating on the young. A similar concentration, apparently permanent, has been established in paediatric medicine (pediatrics); but it should be remembered that this specialty was bitterly opposed when it was first suggested, as paediatric surgery is being opposed at the present time. There is no cause for complaint in this; it is part of the invariable reaction of mankind to new ideas. It is, however, worth examining the arguments against such specialism. No one suggests that children do badly among their contemporaries in institutions specially built, equipped and staffed for them; nor that it is to their disadvantage to be watched continuously by those who have studied their rapid changes of condition. The opposition is from those working in other specialities, who complain that paediatric surgeons are treating cases which "belong" to them. The division of the human body into its systems, each to be treated by a closed corporation dedicated to one of them, is perhaps inevitable given the immense and constantly increasing amount of knowledge to be absorbed and applied. But there are certain disadvantages to this, apart from such obvious ones as the difficulty of deciding whether a diaphragmatic hernia belongs to the specialist in respiratory disease or to him who works in the abdomen. (And what happens to the diaphragmatic hernia patient whose malrotation of the bowel undergoes volvulus post-operatively—if a chest surgeon has operated?—author's note.) One of the most important problems is that when one looks at the patient as a whole—the neurologist, called to a case of spina bifida and hydrocephalus, takes no interest in any deformities of the feet; the orthopaedist leaves the pregnancy history of congenital dislocation of the hip and arthrogrypos to the obstetricians, who respond by ignoring the subsequent history of the child whom they have assisted into the world.

"In order to understand the principles upon which paediatric surgeons work it is most important to realize that they have no ambition whatever to establish another "closed shop" to add to those already in existence; they gladly admit progress in the surgery of the young which comes from those outside their ranks, such as the first successful treatment of oesophageal atresia. And they would also welcome comparisons between their results in such conditions as deformities of the bowel and anus with those gained elsewhere. But as a corollary to claiming no monopoly they also recognize none, and follow their work into any region of the body into which it may lead them."

The necessity for higher standards for the management of infants and children with surgical problems comparable to the achievements in the adult patients has been the stimulus for the establishment of pediatric surgery as a specialty. Although many talented surgeons have contributed significantly to this field, Dr. William E. Ladd was foremost in this country in demonstrating, by his example, the remarkable improvements in patient care that are possible by concentrating the efforts of interested surgeons in the pediatric age group. (This author has operated on 2,000 consecutive patients without a surgical death.) In every aspect of children's surgery to which Dr. Ladd turned his attention, including esophageal atresia and complicated developmental urological problems and neoplasms, remarkably better results followed his efforts. As Dr. Ladd once stated: "The difference between pediatric surgery and adult surgery is quite as great as between pediatrics and adult medicine." Some fifty years ago, Sir Lancelot Barrington Ward, Senior Surgeon of The Hospital for Sick Children in London, stated that, "the adult may be safely treated as a child, but the converse could lead to disaster."

I have been asked, "What is pediatric surgery?" The answer is—"Surgery of patients in the pediatric age group." For many years, the medical problems of infants and children have been recognized as differing extensively from the medical diseases of adults. It is surprising that pediatric surgery has been so slow in developing since the common problems and certainly the developmental congenital problems have very little relationship to the surgical problems of adults.

The author, having a dual background in both pediatrics and pediatric surgery, wishes to emphasize the important position of the practitioner, be he pediatrician or general practitioner, in the handling of the pediatric surgical patient. As this book will verify, his knowledge must be extensive if the patient is to survive. He plays a vital role, if not the most important part, in the ultimate smoothness of the child's course. This is not to downgrade the importance of the technical procedure and the ancillary care during surgery. But it is the practitioner who must first of all suspect the diagnosis; must often prepare the patient for surgery and is usually relied upon heavily in the vital post-operative period. He is also the "child's doctor" and is, therefore, the one who must communicate with anxious parents.

The busy house officer, pediatrician and/or surgeon with the responsibility of handling the pre and post-operative maintenance of the newborn or the small child undergoing surgery needs immediate basic references to help with the frequent problems encountered.

Since the vast majority of pediatric surgery done in this country is performed by general surgeons, and since many of the conventional medications and routines applicable to medical pediatrics are not at all applicable to the pediatric surgical patient, it is imperative that the pediatrician, general practitioner, and surgeon have readily at hand information regarding non-operative aspects of care for the pediatric surgical patient.

The purpose of this book will be to provide this information in an easy-to-read, logical manner. The scope will cover the most important and most frequent pitfalls in pediatric surgical care. Avoidance of errors that lead to an unsuccessful outcome but adequate surgery will be the goal.

On several subjects (notably Hirschsprung's Disease), it is impressive to find that what appears to be marked differences in opinion are not so marked when more deeply probed. In some instances, concepts are at variance because of fundamental differences, but more often because of less basic disagreement as in choice of procedure or timing of surgery. Part of this book will be devoted to the presentation of the varying viewpoints on certain non-operative topics. The training and experience of the surgeon, facilities available, anesthesia, ancillary help, and other matters must be weighed in choosing method of treatment. It is hoped that this presentation will make such choices less hazardous for the individual physician faced with decisions.

Since I have the advantage of general pediatric training (Board Certified in Pediatrics) as well as General Surgical Training and Pediatric Surgical Training (Board Certified in Surgery) (Member of Surgical Section, American Academy of Pediatrics), this book will reflect my training and experience in both fields. Emphasis will be placed on the focal points in diagnosis, and specific methods of treatment.

It is hoped that this book will serve as a personal visit to the workshops of The University of Rochester; Boston Children's Hospital, Harvard Medical School; and The Children's Hospital of Philadelphia, University of Pennsylvania, and will accurately reflect the attitudes and methods of approach of their surgical staffs.

I am indebted to Mr. Milton Burroughs of the Department of Medical Illustration, Medical College of Georgia, for the illustrations, and to my wife, Helen Owings, and my secretary, Mrs. Velma Caldwell, for their help in the preparation of this book.

RICHARD S. OWINGS, M.D.

CONTENTS

		Page
Introduction		*vii*
Chapter		
1.	INCIDENCE OF PEDIATRIC SURGERY	3
2.	THE NEED FOR MORE REGIONAL TOTAL CARE CHILDREN MEDICAL CENTERS	6
3.	SURGERY OF THE NEWBORN	11
4.	FLUID AND ELECTROLYTE REPLACEMENT IN THE OPERATIVE NEWBORN	13
5.	FLUIDS AND ELECTROLYTES	19
6.	BODY METABOLISM DURING STARVATION AND DURING TRAUMA	28
7.	COMPLICATIONS AND THEIR PREVENTION	31
8.	BIOCHEMICAL AND PHYSIOLOGICAL REACTIONS OF THE NEONATE TO SURGERY	36
9.	RESPONSE OF THE CHILD TO SURGICAL STRESS	42
10.	HORMONAL FLUCTUATION IN PEDIATRIC SURGERY	46
11.	PROBLEMS IN ANESTHETIZING A PREMATURE INFANT	50
12.	THE NEONATE'S RESPONSE TO ANTIBIOTICS—USES AND ABUSES	56
13.	BURNS	64
14.	CANCER IN CHILDHOOD	69
15.	TRACHEO-ESOPHAGEAL FISTULAS	94
16.	LYE INGESTION	96
17.	SIMILARITY BETWEEN PATIENT WITH DIAPHRAGMATIC HERNIA AND OMPHALOCELE	98
18.	DIAPHRAGMATIC HERNIA	100
19.	OMPHALOCELE	102
20.	MUCOVISCIDOSIS	104

21. MECONIUM ILEUS   106
22. PEPTIC ULCER   108
23. MISCELLANEOUS SUBJECTS:
     Respiratory Distress Syndrome   111
     Pediatric Surgical Maxims   111
     Intra-uterine Surgery   114
     Comments on Cyanotic Congenital Heart Disease in
        Infancy   116
     Intersex   118
     Neonatal Hypoglycemia   118
     Cysto-urography   119
     Care of the Tracheostomy   122
     Hernias, Hydroceles and Undescended Testicles   123
     Congenital Hypertrophic Pyloric Stenosis   124
     Exstrophy of the Bladder and Cloaca Problems   125
     Hirschsprung's Disease   126
     Intussusception   128
     Imperforate Anus   130
     Oxygen in the Newborn   131
     Mechanism of Tumor Angiogenesis   132
24. LIFE LINE: TOTAL PARENTERAL NUTRITION IN INFANTS WITH
     CATASTROPHIC GASTROINTESTINAL ANOMALIES   135
Index   139

NONOPERATIVE ASPECTS

OF

PEDIATRIC SURGERY

Chapter 1

INCIDENCE OF PEDIATRIC SURGERY

The following comments are based on experience from a number of different sources but primarily concern the percentage of surgical patients that are 15 years or under. At the University Hospital, associated with the Medical College of Georgia, 60% of the admissions are surgical in nature. A review by C. Marshall Lee (Ref: 27th Report of the Ross Pediatric Research Conference, page 11), of all the claims by the John Hancock Life Insurance Company, 25% of the surgical claims were for patients 15 years and under. From this same study, it was noted that 68% of operations in the pediatric age group involved hospitalization, whereas 32% were on an out-patient basis. However, one should note that over the past twenty years there has been a relative decrease in medical admissions and accidental injuries has moved up to the number one killer in pediatrics. From the information compiled by Lee which includes the results of 13 Children's Hospitals, it was found that medical admissions in pediatrics represent 45% and surgical admissions represent 42.5%. Tonsillectomies are not included—constituting some 7½% of pediatric admissions. From children's services in general hospitals, medical cases on pediatrics represented approximately 50% and surgical cases 33%. In Lee's report, one of the problems of the pediatric surgeon is that of remuneration. In the insurance claims reviewed, it is shown that although 25% of the operations in the series were within the pediatric age, they represented only 15% of the surgical charges. A notation is made of the fact that on individuals under 15 years of age, there is a 22% lower than average compensation for surgery as compared with comparable work performed on adults. This is over and above the fact that children are born to the young adults who frequently do not have any insurance coverage and are not financially established. Therefore, the report reviewing insured cases does not take into account a large volume of cases done on the uninsured. Neither is there an accounting of those infants with congenital anomalies disallowed under insurance coverage and infants who require surgery before reaching the age of beginning coverage under certain plans. It is also important to remember that the young father—already confronted with a large hospital bill and obstetrician fee—whose child is born with a surgical problem—finds the situation financially overwhelming. Most pediatric surgeons, realizing these factors, charge such a patient a fee smaller than would normally be expected.

ONE ASPECT THAT NEEDS REVIEW

Pediatrics divorced itself from Internal Medicine in the early thirties and, within a relatively short period, solved many of the major then-existing causes of mortality. Pediatrics could be referred to as "Pediatric Medicine." Pediatric Surgery, however, which has fully as many subtleties in diagnosis and care, has not received the support of the pediatricians that the full potential of the specialty warrants. Pediatricians in general have a very good record in the diagnosis of surgical conditions but following this point of accomplishment the excellence decreases.

Often, the child has the proper diagnosis, the technical aspects of the surgery are properly performed—but the non-surgical aspects of the case are left to chance. An added factor—rather than taking an aggressive stand to see that the newborn with a problem is guided into the care of someone who has the best pediatric surgical experience, the pediatrician confronted with a neonatal problem will often merely ask the parents "who is your surgeon?" The answer would never include a pediatric surgeon who is not a "family surgeon." The physician who has the most training in the specific field concerned should be the best choice. The duty of the pediatrician, therefore, should be to expose his patient to the best possible care. Another point is that one who deals with children entirely has the obligate empathy with the child and appreciates the extreme desirability of avoiding pain and fearful situations.

Along this line, Jeffner and Kaplan reported disturbed reactions in 26 of 60 children between age $1\frac{1}{2}$ and 13 years following hospitalization for tonsillectomy and adenoidectomy. A common experience with young children and toddlers is that they revert to more infantile behavior such as enuresis, fecal soiling, thumb sucking, etc., following hospitalization and particularly following surgery. These reactions do occur frequently and often precipitate more long-lasting disturbances. General practitioners and pediatricians are often remiss in suggesting elective operations even when clearly indicated because of old taboos which do not take into account the increasing safety of anesthesia and armamentaria at the disposal of the anesthesiologist in the form of medications and local anesthetics for minor procedures to decrease the anesthetic risk. The over-avoidance of surgery—of delaying surgical procedures to the detriment of the patient—is often seen and can be of serious consequences.

Pre-operative orientation of the patient and the parent is especially important in allaying fear. Since approximately 60% of the pediatric hospital admissions are children under age 5, it is quite desirable to have rooms with multiple bed areas. Small children can entertain one another for long hours. The parents, when leaving, should make it clear that they are leaving to attend to their home and/or office chores and that they will return at a specific time to reassure the child that he is not being abandoned. As far as possible, children of like ages should be put together and certainly teenagers should have accommodations suitable to their age level and needs. Pamphlets regarding forthcoming hospitalization are no substitute for personal discussions with the parents for preparation. The child is usually far more intelligent than given credit for and will appreciate a straight-forward, completely honest explanation of his problem and forthcoming hospitalization.

Suggested Reading

Lee, C. Marshall: 27th Report of Ross Pediatric Research Conference.

Chapter 2

THE NEED FOR MORE REGIONAL TOTAL CARE CHILDREN MEDICAL CENTERS

There is no better investment than that of properly preparing our young people medically and mentally for the future.

The pablum of increased knowledge has been nurtured by the lawfully wedded parents—need and demand. Increased knowledge has stimulated growth in the fields of child care. To meet the demand for better child care, more trained men and facilities are so badly needed.

Although there are 7 children's medical centers in the Northeast United States in which there is total hospital and out-patient care, special research facilities, and the very important follow-up clinics, there is no one total children's facility in the entire Southeast. There are now 70 million youngsters in the United States 20 years or younger. In the 1970's there will be 90 million in this age category. General hospitals are unable to give total care for the needs of the juvenile or child patient let alone special problems such as newborn deformities and adolescent psychiatric problems. A child has no place in an emergency area where the results of violence among adults is treated. These areas only terrorize the child. Similarly, to place adolescent children in adult wards is poor medicine.

The great number of children in the vast Southeast, larger than most countries, have access only to general medical centers—medical centers geared to helping adults.

Nowhere can the child turn for the consistent total special treatment a child needs.

Nowhere can pediatricians learn and work where the complex equipment required for creating the whole child is centered.

Nowhere can the specialists in children's mental and physical handicaps pool their knowledge and skills, and conduct their research.

6

It's *nowhere* for the children and for those who must bring them into manhood and womanhood.

Children have diseases, physical difficulties, mental disturbances, sensitivities and troubles that are all their own.

No one person can know them all, or even a fair part of them.

They must pool their knowledge and their findings, meet constantly, even hourly, record their findings, catalog them, teach them, invent, devise, discover.

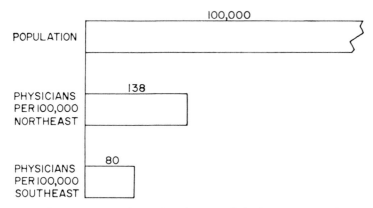

Greater distances and an increasing shortage of physicians available for care in the Southeast make streamlining and pooling essential for better utilization of physician and paramedical facilities

An increasing percentage of graduating physicians are being attracted to non patient aspects of medical care.

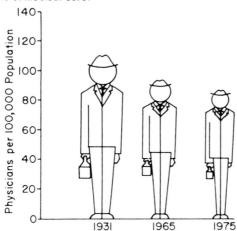

The proportion of physicians available for care of the sick is decreasing. The greatest shortage is seen in the Southeast in child and juvenile care.

Chart 1. Physician to population ratios.

YOUNGSTOWN STATE UNIVERSITY
LIBRARY
323779

PHYSICIANS PER 100,000 CIVILIANS IN EACH STATE

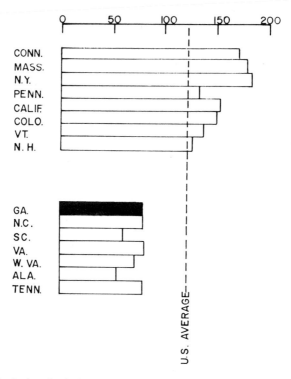

1. The broken line indicates the national average of 138 physicians per 100,000 population.

2. The Southeastern states average 80 doctors per 100,000 population - 58% of the national average.

Chart 2. Physician to population ratios by state.

They must do this in one place. There is no other way.

If they don't they can offer only their single energies and knowledge to the child. And that's not enough.

It's not enough, nearly enough, if that child is our future.

As any parent knows, the child is a man or woman tomorrow. It doesn't take long.

And it doesn't take long to regret the things done wrong and the things that were never done when the man grows into only a part of a man and the woman into only a part of a woman.

Oh, that something might have been done. Or had we known. Or it was known, but the knowledge and skill were nowhere

Time differences in adult care versus child care per physician in the Southeastern states.

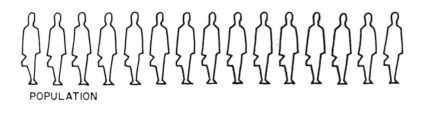

POPULATION

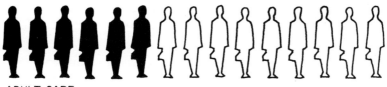

ADULT CARE

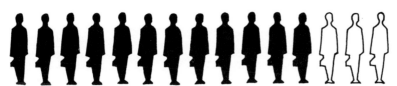

CHILD CARE

Children require twice the number of visits per year compared with adults. Since the physician to population ratio in the Southeast is only 58% of the national average child care suffers disproportionately.

Chart 3.   Physician time requirements.

to be found—outside of Boston, New York, Philadelphia, Baltimore or some other large center.

The children of today must be stronger and wiser adults tomorrow. On this our whole society depends.

The failure to help the child is a personal failure. It is just as much a failure of society.

The most important part of a children's medical center would be the patient.

Emphasis would be on the individual child, not merely toward prolonging life but also toward improving the quality of the child.

This would involve mental and physical hygiene, cure and prevention of disease, child training and all the other complications and necessities for raising the child to be an asset to society and a joy to the parents.

But this also involves the steady, creative effort not so easily dramatized—the education of specialists, the symposiums for dissemination of knowledge, the training of technicians, the establishment of a special library, that constant seeking of new truths —research.

All these and more to be centered where there is already an advancing center of medical knowledge, where transportation and facilities already exist and are expanding, where the intellectual atmosphere and the spirit of the community invite it.

Suggested Reading

Owings, Richard S.: *Brochure: Need for More Regional Total Care Children Medical Centers,* Medical College of Georgia Press.

Chapter 3

SURGERY OF THE NEWBORN

The author has operated on 2,000 consecutive patients without a surgical death. This series includes several patients who had cardiac arrest; all were resuscitated without serious sequelae.

The infant with a serious, life-threatening problem requiring surgery needs adequate oxygen and warmth. He must be handled as little as possible—and any manipulation should be gentle and staged (spaced) to avoid further exhaustion.

The dictum of "intelligent neglect" is a good one: "*observe but do not handle.*" Respiration and pulse are taken gently in the Isolette on an hourly basis. No blood studies are taken—the danger of manipulation being greater than the need for the information sought unless urgently indicated. Micromethod determinations of blood chemistries and blood gases mean less handling of the infant, since only a heel stick is required. If arterial or venous catheters are in place, small amounts of blood can be obtained from them for serial sample monitoring.

The surgery planned is staged so as to allow rest for the infant: the Isolette incubator is kept at 90 degrees fahrenheit with 40% oxygen and high humidity. After initial examination of the infant, a two-hour period is given for the infant to rest. A cutdown is then done exposing only one of the lower extremities; fluids are started at 8 cc/hr. or faster, depending on fluid needs. The infant is again allowed to rest for several hours. Sheet wadding is then placed around all extremities to preserve heat—followed by another rest period. Plasma and Type "O" blood are on call for the baby and are left out to warm.

The infant is placed on the operating table on the "pan" from the Isolette and external heat is maintained. The stomach is vented with a #12 French Catheter with 3 holes to allow for escape of swallowed air and decrease the chance of aspiration as

11

well as to give extra thoracic space for breathing. After a very brief "prep" of the abdomen, the RUQ is infiltrated with ½% procaine, ½% xylocaine and the infant rapidly draped. An Anesthesiologist is on a standby basis—hopefully for oxygen administration only. The intraperitoneal cavity is injected with 20 cc of ¼% procaine and, after a 5-minute waiting period, the abdomen is opened. Exploration is gently performed. All irrigating solutions and towels are warm and the simplest appropriate procedure is performed. Exploration is limited to one hour. The infant is then re-introduced into a warm Isolette incubator.

Post-op monitoring of pulse, respiration and temperature are taken at regular, one-hour intervals and are as gentle as possible. The dictum of "intelligent neglect" is re-emphasized to the nurses—the baby is to be handled only at stated intervals and then as little as possible.

The surgeon should think out the operation carefully and perform the procedure expeditiously. With proper attention to detail, the infant should come off the table with a temperature of at least 96 degrees by rectum. The temptation to attempt everything that can be accomplished technically should be avoided, as survival often hinges on the brevity of surgery and limitation of manipulation.

Chapter 4

FLUID AND ELECTROLYTE REPLACEMENT IN THE OPERATIVE NEWBORN

The busy House Officer, Pediatrician, General Physician and/or Surgeon with the responsibilty of handling the pre- and post-operative fluid and electrolyte maintenance of the newborn needs an immediate method of thinking, based on solid ground, which will help him with the main problems encountered.

The conventional 2½ oz per pound of body weight, or 165 cc/kg, which the general pediatrician uses in replacement of the dehydrated medical pediatric patient (who may have had great G.I. fluid losses) does *not* apply in the I.V. fluid replacement for the operative newborn patient.

In the infant who has had surgery, fluid losses are rarely copious and metabolic demands are of a basal nature. The fact that the insensible loss of the newborn is frequently reduced considerably by the use of 100% saturation in incubators, further diminishes the fluid requirements.

The following factors are worth noting:

(1) Upper intestinal obstruction often accompanies prematurity. In 50% of the patients with high intestinal obstruction, there is also associated icterus. By contrast, infants with low intestinal obstruction do not have either of these problems usually.

(2) The newborn with high intestinal obstruction at birth generally has a 5–10% sodium and chloride deficit and a 5% water deficit, probably resulting from intra-uterine emesis.

(3) Ileus is transient following abdominal surgery in the newborn. Therefore, alimentation can generally be restarted fairly soon. An exception to this is in the case of high intestinal obstruction with associated markedly over-distended bowel.

(4) The smaller the infant—the longer it will take to establish an adequate daily oral fluid volume intake, as well as an iso-

13

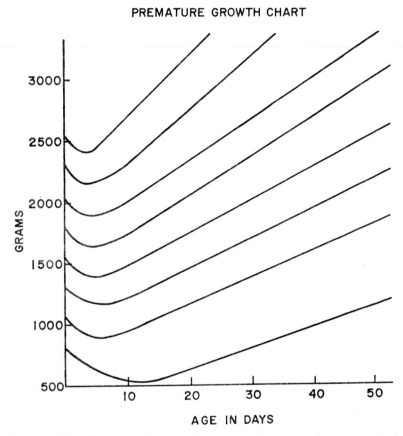

Chart 4. This illustrates the fact that the smaller the infant at birth the longer it will take him to regain his birth weight. The 1000 gram baby may take 20 days to have sufficient fluid and calorie intake to regain his birth weight.

caloric intake. As evidenced by the Belview Weight Chart, it is not uncommon for the 2 lb. infant to take as long as 2 weeks to reach a sufficient fluid and calorie intake to establish weight gain.

(5) It is not uncommon, therefore, in the handling of small infants, to allow an infant to go 24–72 hours before any intake is started. In infants under 3 lbs. or 1500 kg, it is wise to test the "gag reflex" to be sure the infant is able to swallow and, if in doubt, one should use gavage feedings.

(6) The newborn has a larger proportion of body water

located extracellularly; 45% of the fluid compartment is interstitial, as compared with 15% in the adult.

(7) When *abnormal loss of water* from the body occurs, plasma volume is maintained almost entirely at the expense of interstitial fluid. When water volume is excessive, this results in expansion of the interstitial fluid compartment causing edema.

(8) The major ion in the blood vascular space and interstitial space is sodium, therefore, when tissue tugor is poor it connotes inadequate sodium replacement.

(9) An understanding of lean weight water content is important. For every gram of protein, there is an accompanying 4 cc of water. By contrast, for every gram of fat there is only 0.1 cc of water. From this, one sees that the obese infant may become dehydrated much more subtly than one with a lower fat content.

WATER, SODIUM AND POTASSIUM REQUIREMENTS

In the first post-operative days, there is considerable repression of urinary excretion. This is associated with a rather marked anti-diuretic effect and water retention. Added to this, the insensible loss of a newborn may be considerably reduced by the use of 100% saturation in enclosed incubators. The term infant normally excretes about 50 cc of urine in the first 24 hours and by the seventh day this is up to 150 cc.

The basal rates of insensible water loss by the lungs and skin average 100–1200 cc per square meter per 24 hours and since the average infant is approximately 0.2 square meters he would rarely require, in replacement, more than 200 cc I.V. per 24-hour period. This is, of course, unless there have been excessive losses.

Not only does the newborn have considerable repression of urinary excretion during the first days of life, but there is also a tendency for sodium retention and, the well known newborn's difficulty to deal with a sodium load. It may take the newborn several days to excrete a sodium load since very little sodium or potassium is excreted in the first days of life. Although the newborn's sodium level will average 137–138 mEq/liter, the absolute sodium content of the infant per square meter is considerably higher than that of the adult.

The normal newborn plasma concentration of potassium is considerably greater than that of the adult and may range upward to 9 mEq/liter. The infant retains potassium 3–4 times in excess of the amount needed for protein synthesis. In addition to excreting very little potassium in the first days of life, the potassium-nitrate ratio in the urine is identical to that of lean muscle metabolism so there is very little potassium-cellular shift. From these statements, one can conclude that in the first 3–4 days of life—should I.V. fluids be necessary—5% glucose or 5% G/.2% saline is all that is necessary unless there are unusual G.I. losses.

Charts used by surgical services in children's hospitals for I.V. fluid replacement emphasize the dictum "keep the infant dry." This consists of giving basal water replacement of 30 cc per pound per 24 hours; or 65 cc per kg per 24 hours; or 1000 cc per square meter per 24 hours. The newborn infant has a body surface of between 0.2 and 0.25 square meters; therefore, these three calculations are approximately the same.

Daily weights, accurate measurement of urinary output, and BUN levels are three good indicators of the state of hydration. A normal BUN usually connotes an adequately hydrated infant.

The plasma protein concentration in the infant is normally lower than that of the adult and this level drops very rapidly following major surgery—and may be associated with hemo-dilution. But whatever the cause, plasma infusions are of the greatest use post-operatively. Newborns subject to major G.I. surgery frequently require 50 cc of plasma diluted by 50 cc of 5% glucose as a part of their replacement. Infants appear to be able to metabolize infused plasma much more rapidly than adults.

Depletion of sodium leads to a shock-like state and this would be much more frequent if the blood volume were not maintained regardless of the drop in osmolarity. *The principles then in fluid and electrolyte management of the operative newborn are:*

(1) *Not to over-hydrate:* A typical routine for the operative term infant would be to give 8–10 cc of replacement fluid per hour for 24 hours leading to approximately 200–240 cc per 24-hour period.

(2) *The intake-output should be checked at 2-hour intervals and totaled every 8 hours:* Excessive G.I. losses are most unusual in the early post-operative days following neo-natal surgery. 5% glucose or 5% glucose and 1/4% saline is all that is generally necessary for I.V. maintenance. Beginning the second post-operative day, 100 cc of this fluid may be composed of 50 cc 5% glucose and 50 cc of plasma mixed.

(3) *Avoid metabolic acidosis and metabolic alkalosis:* In either condition, if adequate urinary output is established with coloid, the milder of these conditions may be handled by 5% glucose in half normal saline—keeping in mind again that the newborn excretes very little potassium or sodium and handles a sudden load of either ion poorly.

Metabolic alkalosis in the infant is caused by one or two things; either by hypertherapy (especially excessive bicarbonate administration) or, more commonly, by prolonged gastric loss either from suction or vomiting. The prime problem in metabolic alkalosis is one of chloride and potassium loss and the prime effort at correction is that of replacement of chloride and potassium. In the milder varieties of metabolic alkalosis, when good urinary output exists, half normal saline with potassium in the amount of 4 mEq/100 cc is adequate for replacement. Ringer's Lactate which contains 130 mEq sodium/L and 104 mEq chloride/L and 4 mEqL potassium may also be used. In the more serious cases, Darrow's Solution which contains 35.7 mEq/potassium/liter may be used; or, more rarely, ammonium chloride solution.

There are times when the volume of fluid required with the standard I.V. solutions are too voluminous. In these cases, it is wise to use some of the quadrate salts and to give the proper milleqvalents of the ion needed in a more concentrated form. In the more serious degrees of metabolic alkalosis, in which case the CO_2 may be over 40 and the chlorides severely depressed, one may use either Darrow's solution or ammonium chloride solution. If one uses ammonium chloride solution, the calculation is 1 cc per kilogram of body weight to lower the CO_2 by 0.43 milleqvalents/liter—keeping in mind that infants with an elevated CO_2 and elevated BUN often have impaired livers and metabolize ammonia poorly.

When correcting the milder type of acidosis in which there is normal urinary output, the replacement can generally be achieved with Ringer's Lactate or half normal sodium chloride. For more difficult cases, one gives $\frac{1}{6}$ molar sodium lactate in quantities of 4.4 cc/kg and this will increase the CO_2 1 milleqv/kg of body weight. Sodium bicarbonate solution is also widely used for correcting acidosis, usually according to serial blood pH determinations. Formula 1–3 mEq/kg/day.

Based on the Darrow-Yennet concept, it can be seen that the

various body fluid compartments are essentially isotonic and iso-osmotic, with plasma and with each other. It has been demonstrated that water introduced by mouth or I.V. rapidly distributes between the extra and intra-cellular fluid compartments and similar introductions of sodium and chloride will reach a relative osmotic equilibrium rather rapidly. Based on this concept, when ion deficits have existed as in chloride and potassium deficits in metabolic alkalosis and in cases of decreased alkali reserve reflected by a decreased CO_2 level in metabolic acidosis—one may generally replace, thinking of 70% of the body weight as water. For example, in a 3 kg infant, water content equals approximately 2 liters or 2 kg. The deficit of the individual ion is calculated on this fluid volume and $\frac{1}{2}$ of the necessary ion for replacement is given. This replacement is followed by a re-check of the level of correction achieved, at intervals.

In a case of metabolic alkalosis in the same 3 kg infant whose serum chloride if 75, reflecting a 30 mEq per liter drop, a total of 60 milleqv of chloride to correct the 2 liters of fluid content is needed. First, replace 30 mEq of chloride and then re-check. Similarly, the potassium deficit must be replaced. The K & Cl. deficit associated with metabolic alkalosis are extremely interdependent. Both deficits must be corrected simultaneously.

Whereas the above comments have to do with short-term postoperative fluid therapy, it is appropriate to mention that long-term maintenance "total parenteral alimentation" (T.P.A.) is receiving emphasis currently. Previously-disastrous congenital defects are being corrected and salvaged now, leading to a need for prolonged hyperalimentation with weight gain in the infant.

Suggested Reading

Talbert, Nathan B.: *Fluid & Electrolytes: Metabolic Homeostasis,* Harvard Univ. Press. Boston, Mass.

Barnett, H. L.: *Pediatrics,* 15th Ed., Chap. 32, p. 1908, Appleton, Century, Croft, 1972.

Chapter 5

FLUIDS AND ELECTROLYTES

Neonatal plasma contains more chlorides and potassium and less bicarbonate and proteins than the plasma of the older child or adult. When salt depletion predominates over water depletion, the reduction in volume is most striking in the extracellular compartments. This leads to poor tissue turgor. Poor tissue turgor, therefore, denotes salt depletion. The intra-cellular volume is more severly reduced when water depletion predominates.

Water content per kilogram of body weight is much higher in the newborn but this diminishes early in the neonatal period and reaches adult levels at 9 months of age. The infant at this time has a high fat content. Fat is almost water free. The newborn infant loses water out of proportion to solids in the first two or three days. The more immature the infant the more dramatic is this water loss.

The body fluids consist of electrolytes and other substances including glucose, amino acids, and creatinine. Except for a relatively small quantity of water formed in the process of oxidizing carbohydrates, fats and proteins in the body (about 200 cc per meter square per 24 hours), we are almost totally dependent upon exogenous water for maintenance. Under conditions of fasting, an additional 120 cc per meter square per 24 hours endogenous water forms. Obligatory urine water is the smallest volume in which the kidney can excrete waste products.

The infant requires a maximum of 16 mls per milliosmol excreted whereas the adult requires 50 mls per milliosmol. Water loss by way of the lungs and skin is higher in infants, averaging, 1200 mls per meter square per 24 hours. In adolescents and adults, the average is 700 mls per meter square per 24 hours.

The rate at which water is lost from the skin and lungs may be reduced to almost zero when the humidity is raised to 100%

saturation (as in Isolettes). Lowering the ratio of water to solids in body fluids below 3.5 ml per milliosmol results in thirst and concentration of urine, with a tendency to olliguria and fever. In such cases, serum sodium concentration may be elevated to 170 and the serum chloride to as high as 130 mEq/liter. The elevation of water solute ratio in body fluids to above 4 mls/milliosmol is apt to result in headache, fever, and confusion, convulsions and muscle cramps. These symptoms of water intoxication are a result of either an absolute gain in water or absolute loss of solutes. (Reference: Page 15, *Metabolic Homeostasis.*)

Urinary concentration ability may suffer when cellular potassium is depleted. Minimal urine volume varies directly with the rate of solute output, and amounts to approximately 275 mls per meter square in 24 hours in the fasting state. In patients with exceptionally high solute output (burns and severe trauma), the urine volume required may amount to from 2000 to 3000 mls per meter square per 24 hours.

Renal function is immature at birth. Neonates have less ability to diurese but this improves after 4 weeks of age. Neonates also have a larger water surface loss per square meter per 24 hours. In prematures, this surface loss is marked. In the premature, the minimal water required is 1.6 liters per square meter per 24 hours. The adult minimal requirement is about 700 cc to 1 liter per square meter per 24 hours.

Newborn infants have 35% more sodium per kg of body weight than a one year old infant and about 65% more than the adult. Paradoxically, however, serum sodium levels are lower due to the greater relative water content of the newborn. Sodium homeostatis plays a major role in maintaining vascular volume. A decrease in the body sodium results in a dimunition of the extracellular solute content and therefore tissue turgor decreases. To maintain water solute ratio, 7.2 ml of extracellular water is required for each milliosmol of sodium lost. As extra-cellular fluid diminishes, circulatory collapse is prevented to a degree by a transfer of water from interstitial and intra-cellular compartments to the vascular compartments. A reduction in the size of the vascular bed also occurs. Serum sodium concentrations are an *unreliable* index of body sodium but is an inverse index of water solute ratio of body fluids. A high serum sodium usually means too little water: conversely, a low serum sodium usually means

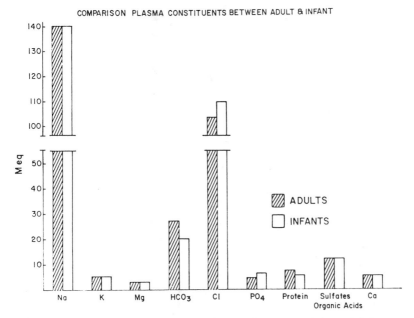

Chart 6. Comparison plasma constituents between adult and infant.

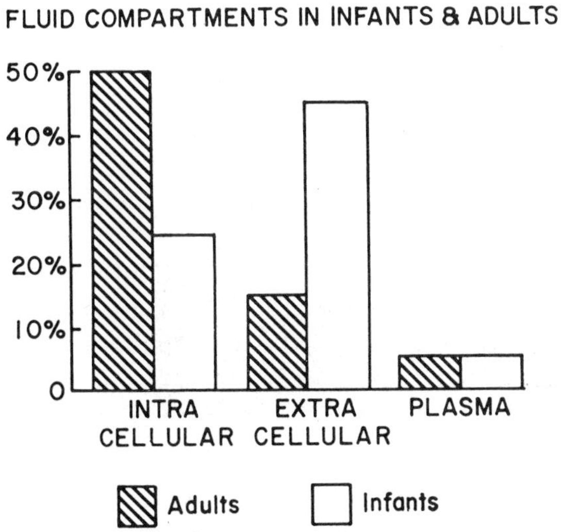

Chart 5. Fluid compartments in infants and adults.

there is a surplus of water in proportion to solutes in the body.

The newborn is unable to handle a sodium load as well as the child or adult. In this connection it is important to remember that tolerances for the human body of amounts of sodium is contingent upon having at least a moderate potassium intake. The body normally contains 45 to 55 mEq potassium per kg of body weight at all ages. The adrenal cortex plays an essential role in allowing the cells to increase their potassium stores temporarily. The body is unable to conserve cellular potassium stores when deprived of potassium unless sodium intake is also restricted. Patients develop cellular potassium insufficiency when maintained on a potassium free, sodium rich solution. Hyperkalemia results in changes in the "T" waves of the EKG. This measurement in Lead 2 is a better index of potassium intoxication than serum levels. Digitalis, by reducing myocardial potassium, may interfere with the use of this as an index. Acidosis may cause a change in the "T" waves which can be confused with the characteristic peaking, as seen with potassium intoxication. If an individual is given large volumes of a high sodium solution which is free of potassium, sodium and hydrogen enter the cell and draw water with it, producing a marked sublevel potassium concentration. The cell function then deteriorates. This may be evidenced clinically by muscular weakness and ileus due to muscle tone loss in the bowel. Other symptoms are loss of urine concentrating ability; lowering or flattening of the "T" wave in Lead-2, and circulatory failure. As referred to earlier, the importance of the sodium and potassium ratio in potassium insufficiency may be difficult to recognize unless the patient has also developed cellular sodium intoxication. Patients who lose hydrochloric acid, as in upper intestinal obstruction with vomiting, lower the concentration of hydrogen ions in the extracellular fluid and develop alkalosis. This, in turn, lessens the ionized calcium and may lead to tetany with convulsions. Cellular potassium depletion usually accompanies this and one will not be able to correct one without correcting both. When the product of the serum calcium multiplied by the serum phosphorus is under 40—tetany with convulsions is imminent.

Magnesium deficiency, while a more subtle entity may also be evidenced by twitching and convulsions. This problem is associated with disorientation of the patient with confusion and bizarre behavior. Lack of correction of the deficiency is ominous. This entity is seen most frequently in a chronically debilitated patient on very little oral intake; and who may also have a chronic fistula.

Correction of the deficiency results in dramatic improvement; failure to correct is associated with extreme restlessness and hyper-irritability and disorientation.

When a patient is on a low-salt diet, the urine becomes salt free. Administration of additional salt causes increased excretion of sodium. High urinary sodium (over 60 mEq/L) in the presence of dehydration, indicates relative adrenal insufficiency. After major surgery, a sodium paradox frequently occurs, in that although there is sodium retention—water retention is greater. Serum sodium levels may be as low as 125 mEq/L. This represents, in part, intracellular movement of sodium with potassium shift in the opposite direction. It also reflects the very active anti-diuretic hormone effect following stress. A patient on no fluid intake (1.7 square meter male) needs 1500 cc for excretory purposes as obligatory fluid loss.

CONCEPTS REGARDING CHEMICAL EQUIVALENTS AND CHEMICAL PRESSURES

Milliequivalents of different elements are unequal in weight but equal in combining power. Talbott has demonstrated that

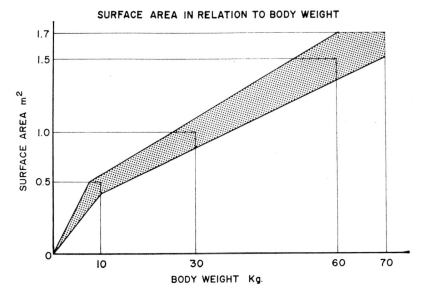

Chart 7. This chart indicates the square meter of body surface to body weight in kilograms.

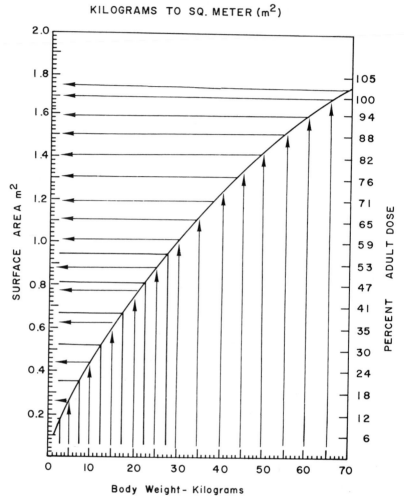

KILOGRAMS TO SQ. METER (m²)

Chart 8. This chart illustrates concisely the relationship of body surface to weight.

requirement turnover rates of fluid and electrolytes are proportionate to body surface area. (Reference: Talbott, Nathan B.: *Metabolic Homeostasis,* Harvard Univ. Press.)

The reasons for not using weight is obvious. To use an illustration of Dr. Harry Statland's (Reference: *Fluid and Electrolytes In Practice,* 2nd Edition, Page 3) "A hostess making up a list of guests for a dance does not invite 1000 pounds of girls and 1000 pounds of boys—rather she is interested that the number of individuals (anions and cations) be equal."

A MOL = one grammolecular weight in grams.

A MOLAR SOLUTION = one grammolecular weight in grams contained in 1000 cc of solution.

TO CONVERT MILLIGRAMS PERCENT TO MILLIEQUIVALENTS PER LITER:

INTAKE OUTPUT

DATE								
ELECTROLYTES								
INTAKE								
Na								
K								
Cl								
OUTPUT								
Na								
K								
Cl								
BODY COMPARTMENTS								
Total Body Water								
Extracellular Volume								
Intravascular Volume								
Plasma Volume								
RBC Volume								
Interstitial Volume								
Intracellular Volume								
Hematocrit								
Hemoglobin								
RBC								
BODY WEIGHT								
SERUM CONCENTRATIONS								
Na (mEq/L)								
K (mEq/L)								
Ca (mEq/L)								
Cl (mEq/L)								
P (mEq/L)								
Total Protein (gm./100cc)								
A/G Ratio								
Urea Nitrogen (mg./100cc)								
CO2								
Urea Clearance (%normal)								
BALANCE SUMMARY								
Water								
Na								
K								
Cl								

Chart 10. Typical progressive intake-output record.

FORMULA: $\dfrac{\text{mg\%}}{\text{atomic wgt.}} \times 10 \times \text{valence} = \text{mEq/liter.}$

MILIOSMOLS: Refers to the osmotic, or pressure effect of a substance.

MILLIEQUIVALENTS: Refers to chemical ionized combining effect.

One mEq of sodium exerts one milliosmol of pressure. However, two mEq of calcium exerts only one milliosmol of pressure. Calcium has the chemical equivalent of two, but only the osmotic force of one particle in solution.

Normal saline has 150 mEq of sodium—how many mEq of chloride is in this solution? ANSWER: 150 mEq chloride, since there is one atom of chloride for each atom of sodium.

How many milliosmols of sodium chloride in this solution? ANSWER: 300 milliosmols of sodium chloride since there are 150 milliosmols each of sodium and chloride.

INTRAVENOUS FLUIDS USED FOR PEDIATRIC SURGERY
(CONTENT PER LITER)

	PLASMA, NORMAL	Saline, Isotonic (0.9%)	Saline, Hypertonic (5.0%)	Darrow's K-Lactate
Na+	142	154	850	122
K+	5			35
Ca++	5			
Mg++	2			
NH4				
Cl-	103	154	850	104
Lactate-	5			53
Citrate-				
HPO4=	2			

	Ringer's Lactate (Hartman's Modified)	Na-Lactate, M/6 (1.9%)	Ammonium Chloride Hypertonic (2.0%)
Na+	130	167	
K+	4		
Ca++	4		
Mg++			
NH+			375
Cl-	111		375
Lactate-	27	167	
Citrate-			
HPO =			

Chart 11. Intravenous fluids used for pediatric surgery.

Blood has 270–285 particles in solution—or 270–285 milliosmols/liter. Saline has 300 milliosmols/liter which is close to the osmolarity of blood and is therefore said to be physiological.

If a solution of Ca Cl$_2$ has 150 mEq of chloride, how many mEq of calcium has it? ANSWER: 150 mEq of calcium. How many milliosmols of calcium chloride? ANSWER: 225 milliosmols—representing 150 milliosmols of chloride and 75 milliosmols of calcium.

Suggested Reading

Talbott, Nathan: *Fluid and Electrolyte Homeostasis,* Harvard University Press.

Moore, Francis D.: *Metabolic Care of a Surgical Patient,* W. B. Saunders & Co.

Statland, Harry: *Fluids and Electrolytes in Practice,* J. B. Lippincott & Co.

Hill, Fontain S.: *Practical Fluid Therapy in Pediatrics,* W. B. Saunders & Co.

Barnett, H. L.: *Pediatrics,* 15th Ed., Chap. 32, p. 1908, Appleton, Century, Croft, 1972.

Chapter 6

BODY METABOLISM DURING STARVATION AND DURING TRAUMA

The three sources of potential fuel in man are carbohydrates, fats and protein. Since fat releases 9 calories per gram it is obviously the most important and also the most abundant source of calorie supply. Carbohydrate in the liver and muscle glycogen supplies energy only during emergencies and is of very short duration. The nitrogen mass of the body is maintained under normal conditions at a peak. Extra calories taken in as dietary protein, despite the "training table" ideas of high protein desirability, are converted into fat and stored as such, not as muscle protein. The same is true of carbohydrates, which if taken in excess since the glycogen depots are also at a peak these calories are rapidly converted to fat and stored as adipose tissue. Thus body nitrogen and carbohydrates are relatively fixed, at a peak level under normal circumstances. Caloric excess or deficiency is met by an increase or decrease in the body's fat mass, and fat serves as man's caloric buffer.

Gamble demonstrated four decades ago that administration of about 100 gm of carbohydrate reduces nitrogen loss in the urine by about 5 times, thus demonstrating the well known "nitrogen-sparing" effect of carbohydrate. How does the patient know metabolically to shut off the amino acid release from muscle and glucose synthesis from these amino acids by the liver? Insulin is the answer. A slight increase in glucose concentration after the initiation of a glucose infusion triggers insulin release which, in turn, inhibits amino acid release from muscle, and amino acid extraction by liver, and gluconeogenesis from what amino acids are extracted. Insulin's primary role is to facilitate glucose uptake into peripheral tissue. Insulin is also very important in maintaining glucose homeostasis by regulating gluconeogenesis as just described.

28

The brain requires gluconeogenically made glucose for fuel. During states of brief starvation gluconeogenesis of the liver produces keto-acids. These cross the blood-brain barrier as does glucose. During prolonged starvation these ketoacids progressively displace glucose oxidation as a source of energy for the brain. The brain goes on a fat fuel by using fatty acids derived from ketoacids. The main effect of this is to spare nitrogen, and urinary nitrogen decreases progressively.

In brief, starvation, insulin, is the signal which decreases protein catabolism and gluconeogenesis. In prolonged starvation, insulin may still be the signal, but a decrease in blood alanine also plays an important role. Of the amino acids coming out of the muscle, alanine and glutamine are the most important.

In prolonged starvation, how does the muscle mass know that the brain can get along on ketoacids, and thereby decrease catabolism of its protein? This control must be at the muscle site in that the circulating level of alanine falls dramatically during this turning off of hepatic gluconeogenesis. Administration of exogenous alanines initiates a prompt hyperglycemia, suggesting the liver to be ready to take more glucose, but the low level of alanine, as set by muscle catabolism, limits the rate of gluconeogenesis. In prolonged starvation, 20–25 gm of protein (3–4 gm nitrogen daily) can allow for several months of survival provided the patient is upholstered with lipid at the start. During this diminution of gluconeogenesis, urea synthesis decreases to two grams or less per day. Since urea is the principle osmotic solute in urine, man may get along on very small volumes of water.

When insulin is lacking, getting back to the careful regulated release of amino acids from muscle or fatty acids for adipose tissue, and the regulated rate of glucose synthesis by liver, these systems go completely unchecked. Muscle releases more and more glucose and, of course, there are more and more ketoacids formed. Glucose levels rise in the muscle and adipose tissue, glucose spills in the urine and there is a profound osmotic diuresis. To check this uncontrolled loss of body calories, the use of insulin and replacing alkali is necessary.

TRAUMA

During trauma there is increased oxygen consumption and this is proportional to the extensiveness of the trauma. There is also accelerated nitrogen catabolism. The brain needs glucose and muscle proteolysis provides the liver with amino acids to make glucose for the brain. The brain adapts to utilization of fat-derived products, further sparing body protein. This is further aided by the administration of 100 gm of glucose per day, as a protein sparing agent. In trauma, there apparently is a reverse of this in that there is selective mobilization of nitrogen and inadequate sparing of nitrogen reserve.

In addition to increased oxygen utilization of the tissue, there is a marked increase of glucose utilization by the polymorphonuclear leucocytes. The fibroblasts also receive their energy by glycolysis. Thus the traumatized patient has a critical need for extra glucose to repair damage. The muscle evidently gets a signal to catabolize amino acids so that the liver can, not only, make glucose for the brain but also for the reparative process. The same is true whether the trauma be that of sepsis or wound formation.

For some reason unknown, the traumatized individual, who is administered glucose does not get the effect of decreasing his protein catabolism. He is even unable to handle exogenous glucose as well and thus the so-called "diabetes" of trauma.

In summary, then, during fasting state, man spares his body protein by excluding glucose utilization as fuel in all tissues capable of using fat. With prolonged fasting, even the brain reduces its glucose requirements by using ketoacids instead. Small amounts of glucose to the briefly-fasted man spares the need for him to make glucose to feed the brain, and thereby spares body protein. In trauma, an extra gluconeogenic load is put on the body apparently to make glucose needed for the reparative process. Glucose administration to the traumatized patient fails to suppress this nitrogen mobilization. The reason for this continued excessive catabolism is not fully understood. This may explain the marked wasting seen in the severely burned patient.

Suggested Reading

Cooke, Robert E.: *The Biologic Basis of Pediatric Practice,* Vol. 1, McGraw-Hill Book Co.

Chapter 7

COMPLICATIONS AND THEIR PREVENTION

There are surgeons who have polished technical ability but who are forever in trouble with their patients and have an abnormally high complication and death rate. Other surgeons who may not appear to be so polished technically, rarely have cases presented at the complication and death conferences because they have learned the key to complications—namely that of prevention.

HYPERNATREMIA

Hypernatremia dehydration is a physiological disturbance that is a true dilemma. It may be seen when an excessive loss of gastrointestional material, from vomiting with or without diarrhea, has occurred. Although there may be an absolute deficit of solute, there is a greater deficit of water. If a hypotonic electrolyte solution is given rapidly, brain swelling is caused by the diffusion of water to the brain being much more rapid than the movement out of electrolytes. Convulsions are commonplace therefore during rehydration. The correction of hypernatremia requires a slow rate of infusion of hypotonic solutions. On the other hand, the inadequate circulating volume makes the use of a slow infusion rather hazardous due to shock. If the concentration of the infusate is increased with electrolytes to enable a speeding of the infusion, then one risks generalized edema and a possible worsening of the hypernatremia.

For a middle-of-the-road course, in the presence of shock, one should first conserve life by the emergency use of a solution containing sodium and colloids in order to restore vascular volume. Five percent albumin or plasma in the volume of 20 cc per kg for infants may be infused fairly rapidly. If there is no shock, the deficit should be calculated and the requirements given slowly over a 48 hour period. A solution should contain 50 mEq/liter of sodium equally divided by carbonate and lactate. After urinary output is established, potassium in the amount of 30 mEq/liter as chloride plus ½ gm of calcium gluconate each 12 hours should be administered. The hydrogen ion status of the patient should be determined and monitored. Should there be a total body excess of salt, peritoneal dialysis with hypotonic glucose (7%) should be undertaken. In evaluating the dilemma, one should remember that convulsions and/or general cerebral edema are not usually fatal, whereas hemorrhage from too great a solid load may have a permanent consequence. Hypertonic solutions although effective in stopping convulsions, are dangerous.

Suggested Reading

Finberg, L.: *Adv Ped, 16*:325–44, 1969.
Ahmed, I.: *Arch Dis Child, 45*:97–103, Feb., 1970.
Pickel, S.: *Pediatrics, 45*:54–9, Jan. 1970.

HYPERTHERMIA

Hyperthermia may be a prime etiologic factor in shock, convulsions and cardiac arrest. Hyperthermia sets up a vicious cycle with loss of fluids, sweating, dehydration leading to additional fever, decreased blood volume and shock. Associated with this, the peripheral vascular bed dilates in an attempt to dissipate heat. Therefore, it is imperative that the temperature (in a patient with a ruptured appendix, for example) be brought down to some reasonable, satisfactory level before anesthesia is instituted. For each degree of temperature elevation, there is an increase in the metabolic rate of 7.2% which in turn necessitates an increase of 5% in the ventilation rate of the body in order to maintain metabolic homeostasis. The cardiac rate increases 5 to 10 beats per minute per degree rise in temperature and heart action becomes inefficient with decreased cardiac output.

Immaturity may contribute to operative hyperthermia through an incompetent central nervous system. For this reason, the febrile child or infant should have every opportunity to dissipate heat by radiation and evaporation. In this regard, one should remember that heat stroke is significantly more common in children.

In summary, maintenance of optimal body temperature is

extremely important in infants and children: they readily develop either hypothermia or hyperthermia during surgery. It is imperative to prevent excessive hypothermia in infants under one year and body temperature should be recorded during the procedure.

Hyperthermia, if allowed to go untreated, leads to an increased metabolic rate; peripheral vascular dilitation; a decrease in the circulatory blood volume with rapid exhaustion and cerebral edema; arrythmias and cardiac arrest.

HYPOTHERMIA

During anesthesia a child, and particularly an infant, loses much of his ability to maintain normal temperature. His temperature tends to fluctuate with that of his environment. Unless vigorous efforts are made to conserve body heat, one is apt to have a cold, cyanotic infant; particularly following procedures in excess of two hours duration during which the viscera has been exposed. The recovery room attendant may report that the temperature of the infant is 94 degrees. This happens to be the low point on the thermometer and the infant's temperature may actually be as low as 90 degrees. The infant is unable to shiver and, thereby, increase his body heat. He has a much larger relative abdominal volume space per unit weight than the older child or adult; and a much larger surface area per unit as well. Whereas hypothermia may have some uses in the older child or adult in particular procedures, it is very dangerous for the infant. During hypothermia the oxygen disassociation curve moves to the left and the infant actually receives far less oxygen than is necessary to maintain him. The use of sheet wadding to insulate the extremities and warm water bags are valuable methods of maintaining external heat which pay great dividends in preventing hypothermia in the infant. Unrecognized hypothermia can inhibit all respiration. Hypothermia leads to depressed respiration, hypoxia and predisposes a baby to arrythmias and ventricular fibrillation. In addition to the proportionately larger surface area per unit of weight, the abdomen is proportionately larger in the infant and the periotoneal surface area is relatively greater. His metabolic needs and respiration rate are greater. Temperature changes will occur very rapidly toward hypothermia unless appropriate preventive measures are instituted.

Hypothermia in the neonate is probably the most common

cause of cardiac arrest and shock encountered by the occasional surgeon who is unfamiliar with this very vital need to conserve heat during surgery in the newborn.

Suggested Reading

Silverman, Wm. A.: Influence of Temperature on Metabolism in the Neonate, 49th Ross Conference on Pediatric Research.

PREVENTION OF POST-OPERATIVE ADHESIONS

The incidence of post-op adhesions from intestinal obstruction in infancy is very high. Adhesions are formed from:

(1) Trauma to the intestinal serosa which leads to an

(2) Inflammatory response associated with increased permeability of blood vessels and cell destruction with the

(3) Release of by-products of cell damage followed by protein rich exudate, due to the action of histamine and permeability factors. Some of the accumulated exudate is removed by fibrinolytic activity and re-absorbed but the remaining exudate is transformed by fibroplasia into collagen and then to fibrosis.

The important factors in prophylaxis of intestinal adhesions in addition to gentle surgical technique is to attempt to:

(1) Minimize the inflammatory reaction and to reduce the amount of exudate. This in turn will decrease the amount of fibrosis and

(2) The other approach is to delay fibroplastic organization to allow serosal cells to cover the denuded areas.

For this, drugs are used to prevent adhesions. Promethazine inhibits the vascular permeability and blocks the reaction resulting from nucleosides, peptides and globulins and, in contrast to other antihistamines, it blocks the release of histamine from mast cells. It also protects the lysosome system reducing cellular damage due to release of acid hydrolytic enzymes.

Dexamethasone reduces the exudate phase and limits secondary damage of inflammation. It also inhibits fibroplastic migration, proliferation and organization.

The Promethazine dose in infants and newborns is 0.5 mg/kg q 4 h and the same dose can be given intraperitoneally. The adult dose is 25 mg of Promethazine and 20 mg of Dexamethasone q 24 h. This is given 4 hrs. and 2 hrs. pre-operatively. The same dose

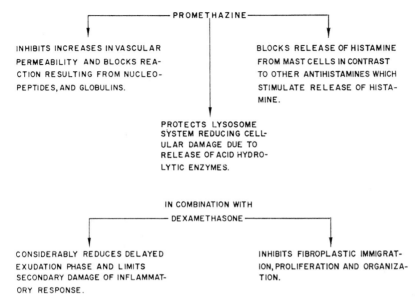

Chart 12. This illustrates the probable mechanism of action of the combination of drugs that have been quite successfully used in preventing post-operative adhesions.

is then given q 4 h for 48 hours after surgery. The post-operative dose is given in 50 cc. of saline intraperitoneally.

Suggested Reading

Brij, M. L. K., *et al.: Arch Surg, 98*:301–4, March, 1969.
Brij, M. L. K., *et al.: Surgery, 65*:629 32, April, 1969.
Moore, T. C., *et al.: Surgery, 67*:364 68, Feb., 1970.
Replogle, Robt. L.: Scientific Exhibit, Am. College Surgeons, 1969.

HEAVY DRAPES

Other frequent preventable complications may be attributed to excessively heavy drapes. A two-pound drape dragging on a five-pound infant's chest is too great a burden for an already marginal infant to carry. Experienced anesthetists have put forth the thought that most infants in this counry are under-ventilated during surgery. Indeed it is very important in anesthesia for the anesthetist to allow the infant to maintain his own respiration in that, without intubation, it is next to impossible to breathe an infant for a long period of time safely. If, added to this, heavy drapes are used, one can predict disastrous results.

Chapter 8

BIOCHEMICAL AND PHYSIOLOGICAL REACTIONS OF THE NEONATE TO SURGERY

The first balance studies that were done on operative newborns and prematures were done by Dr. Peter Paul Rickham of the Alderhey Clinic in Liverpool, England. Much can be learned by a review of his findings.

"During the last five years, we have studied the biochemical changes induced by surgical procedures on newborn infants. Over 600 infants have been investigated by performing studies of serial blood chemistries and making accurate records of intakes. However, because of fluctuations in the blood chemistry occur so rapidly and are often actually misleading, nine infants were selected to be investigated by means of balance studies. Thus it was hoped to develop a pre and post operative regimen based on laboratory as well as clinical information.

"It has been known for some time that neonates differ from older infants and children in their extraordinary resistance to surgical trauma. These studies were undertaken to determine whether there were also differences in their metabolic response.

"The metabolic response of a newborn infant who had repair of an omphalocele on the day of birth and whose fluid and electrolyte balance was undisturbed prior to operation showed a negative nitrogen and potassium balance that lasted only one day after his operation. As soon as there was any oral intake, the nitrogen and potassium balance became positive. During the short negative phase, the potassium:nitrogen excretion ratio was 3.1 mEq/gm, closely approximating the value for lean muscle tissue. As is expected in the neonate, sodium and chloride retention was marked. Although the postoperative fluid output was small, evidencing some water retention, his urinary output was no smaller than that observed in the normal neonate, and water retention

36

was not marked. The infant with pure dehydration prior to operation presents a similar picture.

"These findings are in contrast to those of a newborn infant with intestinal obstruction who had lost both water and electrolytes prior to operation. This infant showed some postoperative fluid retention but his nitrogen balance was persistently negative and large quantities of nitrogen were excreted by the kidneys. The urinary concentration of nitrogen rose to above 1000 mg. percent, demonstrating that the neonatal kidney can excrete nitrogen in a concentration similar to that of adults. The potassium balance also continued to be negative, with large amounts being lost in the urine as well as in aspirated gastric fluid. The potassium: nitrogen excretion ratio was only 2.86 mEq/gm. This means that, in spite of preoperative vomiting and postoperative intestinal suction, no potassium shift occurred as is seen in the adult. Retention of both sodium and chloride was marked.

"The differences between the physiological response to surgery of the infant and that of the adult can be summarized as follows:

"(1) The newborn infant rarely develops an elevated temperature postoperatively.

"(2) Postoperative weight loss, so conspicuous in the adult, is usually absent in the neonate. If it does occur, the infant quickly resumes his preoperative weight.

"(3) Postoperative water retention is not conspicuous in the newborn infant. It is often difficult to assess his state of hydration in the presence of his normally restricted urinary output.

"(4) Increase in nitrogen excretion occurs postoperatively in neonates but is not greater than that found when he is starved.

"(5) A most extraordinary difference is the absence of a potassium shift from the cell to the urine of the infant. In contrast, this shift is very prominent both in the adult and in the older child subjected to surgery.

"(6) Postoperative sodium and chloride retention is common to both, but sodium retention on the day of operation or the first postoperative day is not observed in the neonate.

"Next we attempted to learn the age at which the biochemical response of the neonate to surgery shifted to that observed in the adult. It is well known that the infant more than two weeks of age loses his "resistance" to surgical trauma. At about this same time, his response to those muscle-relaxing drugs whose action depends upon the migration of potassium ions across the cell membrane changes from the typical neonate response to the adult pattern. Three three-week-old infants were studied by balance techniques after operation, and each had a response very similar to that found in the adult. Nitrogen excretion during the postoperative period was marked. Even with considerable postoperative nitrogen intake, the balance remained in the neighborhood of zero. In spite of a considerable potassium administration, prolonged and excessive potassium excretion lasted throughout the whole period of observation. During the negative phase, the potassium:nitrogen excretion ratio was 7.2 mEq/gm, considerably in excess of the potassium:nitrogen ratio in lean muscle tissue. Each infant also showed the typical potassium shift found in the adult subjected to surgery.

"Our investigations, therefore, demonstrate that there is both a quantitative and qualitative difference in the response of the neonate subjected to surgery. This difference is most marked with regard to potassium. McCance showed that the newborn infant's muscle cells contain more potassium than do those of adults. Our infants appeared to have no difficulty in excreting potassium via the urine, and in general their kidney function was extraordinarily good.

"There is evidence that postoperative potassium excretion in the adult is controlled by the adrenal cortex. Corticosteroid and ketosteriod excretion in the urine increases after operation, and the eosinophil count falls, only to rise again above that found preoperatively. In the newborn infant, the adrenal gland is relatively large. Its cortex is mainly fetal in type, with a thin rim of the adult type. Starting on the fifth day of life, the adult zone increases rapidly in size, and by the time the infant is two to four weeks old has differentiated into the zona glomerulosa and the zoma fasiculata: Emery and his collaborators have shown by histochemical methods that the steroid content of the newborn adrenal gland is extremely low, and that disease produces little, if any, histochemical change. Evidence relating to adrenal function in the neonatal period is conflicting, but there appears to be a significant difference in the pituitary-adrenal response to any stress between the neonate and the older child or adult. We have not attempted to determine the corticosteroid levels in our infants. Their eosinophil counts are most irregular, and do not appear to bear any relation to their clinical pictures. By three weeks of age, however, their eosinophil response closely resembles that found in adults.

"There are a number of practical applications resulting from this investigation. The newborn infant has a comparatively undeveloped temperature-regulating center. His temperature tends to fluctuate with the temperature of his environment, and through his relatively large area of body surface, heat loss is rapid. An incubator at 85° F will prevent any marked fall in temperature; but a subnormal temperature does not, in fact, seem to be injurious to the full-term infant. It does not appear to influence metabolism and wound healing adversely. Postoperative weight loss is often surprisingly small in the newborn infant. Over short periods, changes in body weight are the best guides to changes in the patient's total body water and his state of hydration. The newborn infant tolerates starvation well; therefore, it is of no great importance if the calorie intake remains low for several days after operation. On the other hand, infants who are unable to take nourishment by mouth for prolonged periods are difficult to sustain adequately by intravenous infusions, and present a real problem. It is not always appreciated how very small the newborn infant's daily fluid requirement is and how easily he can be overinfused. Fluid requirement and urinary output are especially small during the first days. Postoperative water retention, although not as marked as in the adult, does occur, and further reduces the neonate's fluid requirement. Since laboratory examinations such as the hematocrit or BUN or NPN can be very misleading, the degree of hydration in infants is best estimated clinically.

"The newborn infant withstands water deprivation extremely well and, hence, it is usually unnecessary to replace pure water loss preoperatively. Postoperatively, however, fluid loss must be correctly assessed by measuring gastric aspirations and estimating urinary output. Insensible water loss can be greatly reduced by keeping the infant in an atmosphere of 100 percent humidity. Correct fluid replacement is of great importance in the postoperative period, but it is better to give too little rather than too much. As a rough guide, fluid is given the infant at the rate of a total of 5 ml/hour during the first 24 hours postoperatively, and then 10 ml/hour thereafter. Of course, in the presence of marked dehydration, the amount must be increased. With such small amounts, the quantities of fluid have to be very accurately measured and charted. The hazards of a "run-away" postoperative infusion are such that the sooner the intravenous infusion can be discontinued and oral feeding started, the better.

"Unfortunately, prolonged ileus following abdominal operations is common in neonates (not in the author's experience); for that reason, gastric suction and intravenous infusions often have to be continued over long periods. Although the dangers of intravenous infusions are great, the dangers of vomiting and inhalation of vomitus are even greater.

"The newborn infant catabolized protein for some time after birth, and during this period, any operation increases nitrogen excretion slightly. If the catabolic phase is prolonged more than two or three days, nitrogen replacement by diluted plasma infusion is indicated.

"The newborn infant, whose kidneys have difficulty in excreting salt, is prone to develop edema if he is given intravenous saline following operation. If there has been little or no salt loss, we infuse only 5 percent glucose water. The gastric and intestinal secretions of neonates contain only slightly less sodium and chloride than those of adults, and prolonged gastric suction will cause severe sodium and chloride loss. Should salt have been lost by prolonged gastric or intestinal suction, we give $\frac{1}{5}$ normal saline with 5% glucose by infusion. Only if the salt loss is excessive do we occasionally use small amounts of $\frac{1}{2}$ normal saline.

"As the newborn infant excretes little potassium following operation, it is usually unnecessary to give any intravenous potassium, even after operations requiring gastric suction. Since intestinal juices contain a considerable amount of potassium salts, prolonged intestinal syphonage will, however, produce hypokalemia in the neonate just as it does in adults. Hypokalemia can be prevented by giving 50–60 ml of Darrow's solution intravenously each day to infants who are maintained on gastric suction for longer than three days.

"Actually, very few biochemical tests are of any value in gauging post operative fluid management. Occasionally, a hemoglobin reading or an estimation of the plasma potassium is useful. Determination of blood nonprotein nitrogen, plasma alkali reserve, plasma chloride or protein concentration can be on occasion most helpful. These tests should be performed by a laboratory with 24-hour facilities to undertake analyses using considerably less than 0.5 ml of plasma. No practical value ensues from these tests unless accurate results can be obtained within a few hours.

"My remarks reveal how little is actually known as yet about the many physiological changes initiated by operating on a newborn infant. There is no doubt that, without greater insight into his physiology and those processes by which he adjusts himself to his extrauterine existence, there will be little further progress in this aspect of neonatal surgery."

Suggested Reading

Rickham, P. P.: *The Metabolic Response to Neonatal Surgery,* Harvard University Press, Cambridge, Mass., 1957.

McCance, R. A., *et al.: Arch Dis Child, 29*:104, 1954.

Stoner, H. B., Whiteley, H. J., and Emery, J. L.: *J Path & Bact, 66*:171, 1953.

Christensen, H. N., *et al.: J Biol Chem, 209*:413, 1954.

Smith, C. A.: *Pediatrics, 16*:254, 1955.

Chapter 9

RESPONSE OF THE CHILD TO SURGICAL STRESS

Reaction to surgical stress is an all-inclusive term used to designate those physiological deviations from normal that occur during and following a surgical procedure. Fortunately, the organism can usually adapt to this added stress and maintain its equilibrium. However, the less the total stress imposed upon the individual, the more easily he will recover. Infants and children are immature in their capacities for adaptation. They appear to have a limited reserve, particularly in the respiratory, cardiovascular, renal and endocrine systems.

Because the lung alveoli are not fully developed saccules in infants, a state of relative respiratory insufficiency is present. There is increased oxygen consumption per square meter of surface area. The newborn with a limited tidal volume of 15 to 20 ml will respond to a respiratory stimulus by increasing his rate, already normally rapid, rather than by increasing his depth of respiration. In this instance, an increase in rate is not an efficient response. Although the newborn infant seems to tolerate hypoxia longer and better than adults, diminished oxygenation is a common precursor to cardiac arrest in both groups. This is especially important when the respiratory rate and depth are controlled by the hand of the anesthetist during endotracheal anesthesia. If an infant is hyperventilated, his carbon dioxide tension may be diminished to the extent that apnea results. Apnea may also develop secondary to fatigue of the respiratory musculature. Fatigue may result from heavy drapes, the inherent resistance of anesthetic machines, or partial respiratory obstruction.

An infant has much more cardiac reserve. In the early months of life, his heart does less work than it had done during fetal life, because it no longer propels blood through the cord and placenta. This may explain why infants can tolerate the added load of major operative procedures. But the loss of 30ml of blood represents one-tenth of the infant's total circulating blood volume, and is for the infant equivalent to the loss of 600 ml by the normal adult. Consequently, when small quantities of blood are lost they must be replaced to prevent added stress on his cardiovascular system. The most inefficient segment of the cardiovascular system is the infant's limited peripheral vasomotor control. Since his vasomotor reflex to blood loss is ineffectual, his circulating blood volume must be kept relatively constant.

The renal system of the newborn has a limited reserve. As shown microscopically by a nephrogenic zone in which glomeruli are still developing, anatomic renal maturation is not achieved until an infant reaches approximately five and one-half pounds of weight. Urea clearance studies show that renal function is limited in comparison to that of adults until the child reaches the age of three months. The ability of the kidney to concentrate urine is also limited, and hypotonic urine is normal in infancy. As a result, infants and children withstand both overhydration and dehydration poorly. Likewise, electrolyte balance is precarious and an excessive loss or overinfusion of anions or cations is poorly tolerated. Early recognition of acidosis or alkalosis and early initiation of appropriate therapy are essential.

The infant's endocrine system is incompletely understood. After his third day of life, the normal infant shows a marked diminution of the circulating corticoids from the level that exists at birth, which is comparable to that of the normal adult. The cause of this fall is unknown. Although his response to stimulation by ACTH is sluggish, it probably is adequate in the presence of sufficient stress. With a severe infection, high levels of circulating adrenal corticoids are found. The same response is presumed to follow a major surgical stress.

Methods of minimizing stress to the infant during surgery can be formulated from an understanding of these inadequacies or limitations in adaption. Since hyperthermia taxes the cardiovascular system, a McQuiston-Bigler type mattress should be available to cool the patient as needed. It is also useful to warm the patient should the occasion arise. With its routine use, the mad scramble to get it under the patient with all the drapes in place and the field sterile is avoided.

Body temperature should be continuously recorded throughout the surgical procedure. Other measures include regular aspiration of secretions and continuous monitoring of the heart beat by a stethoscope strapped onto the chest. If the surgeon needs the entire chest exposed, an esophageal stethoscope can be used. A small earphone attached to one ear will allow continuous listening.

After completion of the surgical procedure, usually everyone relaxes. The immediate attention of the anesthesiologist, surgeon and circulating nurse is diverted from the patient. But it is at this time that many patients develop trouble.

Following operation, the responsibility for observing the young-ster is transferred from the anesthetist to the personnel in the recovery room. What are the essential parts of a recovery room? We feel that a close proximity to the operating room has definite, important advantages. The trip between the two is short, and the chance of aspiration or other catastrophe is minimized. In the event of trouble, all the personnel and facilities of the operating room are immediately at hand. Our recovery room is also adja-cent to the doctor's lounge and dressing room which usually has a concentration of available manpower in case of emergency. Rapid communication should be possible between the recovery room personnel and the operating room supervisor, so that the recovery room nurse does not have to dial a phone or run down the hall to obtain assistance.

Recovery room nurses should be trained by the anesthesia department to recognize the sound of a partially obstructed air-way in a child, and in methods of inserting or removing airways and of manipulating the jaw so that the airway remains patent. They are instructed to place unconscious youngsters on their sides rather than on their backs, to minimize the possibility of aspiration. They are able to observe respirations easily because either the patient's chest or abdomen is exposed. If added heat is needed, of course, a pad or hot water bottle can be placed on the child's back.

All equipment in the recovery room should be accessible and maintained in good working order. Oxygen and suction should be available in each subdivision of the recovery room. An equip-ment cart should be available to quickly transport needed items to the patient's bed. Endotracheal tubes, masks, aspirating cathe-ters, small polyethylene tubing for aspirating endotracheal tubes, and a laryngoscope rest in full view on its top. Every morning, one of the primary functions of the recovery room nurse is to make sure that all this equipment is in good working order. In one drawer are various catheters to aspirate the pharynx. In another drawer emergency medications are available. In the bottom drawer sterile sets for thoracentesis, tracheotomy, or cardiac massage are available.

All children who received anesthesia are automatically taken to the recovery room. Once the child responds to minor stimuli, he is transferred to the acute surgical ward. No child leaves the recovery room until he has been re-evaluated by a member of the anesthesia or surgical department.

The acute surgical ward is almost as important to our service as the recovery room. An acute surgical ward allows a concentration of nursing power in a small area where good nursing service is really needed. Six patients immediately post-operative demand far more attention than does a ward of 20 convalescent patients. The nurses learn to handle necessary equipment efficiently. This concentration of experience has led to marked increase in our awareness of the specific problems of nursing care which are involved in such cases as postoperative tracheoesophageal fistula. The house staff, too, can concentrate their attention on the acute surgical unit to review all acutely ill patients very quickly.

By integrating our immediate postoperative care, we have been able to avoid some postoperative disasters. Nevertheless, it should be emphasized that since currently we really don't understand the factors contributing to some catastrophes, our success is far from complete. With adequate investigation this situation should prove remedial.

Suggested Reading

McCance, R. A. and Young, W. F.: *J Physiol, 99*:265, 1941.

Hand, A. M., and Leininger, C. R.: *M Clin North America, 34*:53, 1950.

Bigler, J. A., and McQuiston, W. O.: *JAMA, 146*:551, 1951.

DeBoer, Arthur: 27th Ross Pediatric Research Conference.

Chapter 10

HORMONAL FLUCTUATION IN PEDIATRIC SURGERY

With surgery, there is usually an increase in both plasma and urinary cortiocosteroids; each of the successive stages involved before, during and after surgery include many factors that are able to produce alterations in adrenal function. One possible factor is the level of anxiety in the pre-operative patient. The studies of Sandberg *et al.* Franksson *et al.*, and Viikari and Thomasson have indicated that such anxiety does not significantly elevate the circulating corticoids. In the rhesus monkey, certain types of pre-operative medication, including reserpine and chlorpromazine, have been found to increase the concentration of 17-hydroxycorticosteroids, while others, such as sodium pentobarbital, lead to a decrease. In contrast, other studies have shown that chlorpromazine administration inhibits an adrenal response to hypoglycemia.

Sandberg *et al.*, have observed that, even though plasma concorticosteroid in seven of eight patients following their induction by the general anesthetics, Pentothal, Cyclopropane and Ether, while only one patient undergoing spinal anesthesia showed a similar elevation. Virtue and colleagues found definite increases in plasma corticoid levels in 15 of 35 patients induced with ether. For the group, the mean rise was significant. Neither cyclopropane, nitrous oxide, nor spinal anesthesia produced a significant change. From the time of onset of the actual surgical procedure, the plasma concentration of 17-hydroxycorticosteroids increases rapidly. The levels continue to rise for as long as six to nine hours following the operation, depending upon the length of the procedure. Reece *et al.*, measured the increase of urinary corticoid excretion, comparing patients undergoing herniorrhaphy with those undergoing partial gastrectomy. The average output after herniorrhaphy was 25 mg per day, whereas following gastrectomy it was over 40 mg per day. In the former group the urinary corticoids remained increased over control levels for two to four days, while in the latter they continued at elevated levels for as long as six days. Holman and Migeon have found that in children even a minor surgical procedure produces a sharp rise in both plasma and urinary corticoids, an increase which is more pronounced than that following similar procedures in adults.

It is true that elevated plasma corticoids do not necessarily mean that there has been a more rapid output or secretion of steroids by the adrenal. However, since urinary corticoids are also elevated, it would suggest that the actual production of corticoids is increased. The experimental work of Hume and Nelson in dogs has demonstrated that the concentration of cortisol in the adrenal vein increases during surgery.

Sandberg *et al.*, have observed that, even though plasma concentrations of corticoids rise as high in the postoperative patient as they do in the normal individual following ACTH administration, and additional increment will result in the former group after an injection of ACTH. They also observed that intravenously administered hydrocortisone was not metabolized as rapidly after surgery as it was during control periods. These studies in children have produced similar results. Such evidence would suggest that the increase in plasma corticoids during and following surgery is due to both an elevated cortisol production and a decreased rate of conjugation or excretion of the hormone.

If cortisol were metabolized at a slower rate during surgery, we would expect to find low levels of corticoid conjugates in the blood. Helmreich *et al.*, found the levels of both conjugated and free steroids to be elevated under these conditions. Our studies in children show that the levels of conjugated coritcoids in plasma are certainly not low.

The free or active hormone is known to be loosely bound to protein and thus not freely excreted by the kidney. After conjugation with glucoronic acid in the liver, the hormone becomes water-soluble and is readily excreted by the kidney. If the rate of renal excretion of glucuronides were slower than normal, an increase in the levels of plasma conjugates would result. Depending upon the degree of inhibition of renal excretion, such an increase could be observed even in the presence of a reduced rate of conjugate formation by the liver. We believe that the high levels of conjugated steroids found after surgery in our studies can probably be best explained on the basis of such a decrease in renal excretion.

The mechanism leading to this increase in plasma corticoids following surgery has not yet been satisfactorily explained. One postulate is that toxic metabolites such as histamine are produced as a result of tissue trauma and act directly on the pituitary gland to stimulate the production or release of ACTH. Unfortunately, however, an infusion of 1 mg of histamine induces no such increase in corticoids. Sayers has suggested that the stimulus is provided by the increased utilization of corticoids at the tissue level. The subsequent decrease in circulating corticoids might induce an increase in ACTH production which, in turn, would lead to an increase in corticoid production by the adrenal. Many facts tend to confirm this hypothesis, such as the observation that the administration of exogenous cortisol decreases ACTH production and produces adrenal atrophy. However, it is difficult to explain why an initial increase in the corticoid level, resulting from such a stimulus, does not shut off the whole process immediately. Another valid objection to this theory is the failure to demonstrate any alteration in tissue utilization of the hormone.

Long hypothesized that the stimulus would act directly on the adrenal medulla to release epinephrine which would act on the pituitary gland, directly or via the hypothalamus, to increase ACTH production and thus lead to an increase in circulating corticoids. However, the injection of exogenous epinephrine does not produce any significant change in plasma corticosteroids.

Another postulate is that of Guillemin and Rosenberg who believed that they had detected a chemotransmitter in hypothalamic extracts which would stimulate ACTH production by the pituitary gland, but this material, as yet, remains unidentified. The exact mechanism that leads to increased corticoid levels remains unknown. Similarly, the purpose of this increase is also unclear. Is the negative nitrogen balance associated with surgery produced by increased circulating corticoids? Possibly it is. At the same time, it is known that the Addisonian requires additional exogenous hormone to withstand surgery. Therefore, the paradox of coexisting beneficial and detrimental effects exists. Perhaps future investigation will clarify this enigma.

Suggested Reading

Sandberg, A. A., Eik-Nes, K., Samuels, L. T., and Tyler, F. H.: *J Clin Invest, 33*:1509, 1954.

Franksson, C., Gemzell, C. A., and von Euler, U.S.: *J Clin Endocrinol, 14*:608, 1954.

Viikari, S. J., and Thomasson, B. H.: *Acta Endocrinol, 24*:361, 1957.

Christy, N. P., Knight, M., Langson, D., and Jailer, J. W.: *J Clin Endocrinol, 16*:913, 1956.

Virtue, R. W., Helmreich, M. L., and Gainza, E.: *Surgery, 41*:549, 1957.

Reece, M. W., Edwards, K. M., and Jepson, R. P.: *Surgery, 42*:669, 1957.

Hume, D. M., and Nelson, D. H.: *J Clin Endocrinol, 15*:839, 1955.

Helmreich, M. L., Jenkins, D., and Swan, H.: *Surgery, 41*:895, 1957.

Sayers, G.: *Physiol Rev, 30*:241, 1950.

Long, C. N. H.: *Res Prog Hormone Research, 7*:75, 1952.

Guillemin, R., and Rosenberg, B.: *Endocrinology, 57*:599, 1955.

Mingeon, Claude J.: 27th Ross Pediatric Research Conference.

Chapter 11

PROBLEMS IN ANESTHETIZING A PREMATURE INFANT

The Dean of Pediatric Anesthesiology in the United States is Dr. Robert M. Smith of the Boston Children's Hospital. To quote some of his comments from the literature is most informative.

"The problems that we encounter in anesthetizing premature infants relate principally to the individual physiologic characteristics of the infant and to the type of surgery.

"The vast majority of infants who undergo surgery in the neonatal period do so because of some lesion involving the gastroenteric tract. These lesions may be located intrathoracically, e.g., eventration of the diaphragm or esophageal atresia with tracheo-esophageal fistula or may be located intra-abdominally, e.g., atresia or stenosis of the small intestine, annular pancreas or meconium ileus. It is important to recall that the higher the level of obstruction, in general, the smaller the infants are at birth.

GOALS OF ANESTHESIA

"There are *four fundamental goals* or purposes in anesthetizing surgical patients. These may be considered with regard to our approach to the neonate. The first reason for administering an anesthetic agent is to achieve *analgesia*. The fact that the small infant may lie on the operating table with his viscera exposed for several hours, while he sucks on an airway, suggests we need worry *very little about pain control in premature infants*. A second consideration is to produce *hypnosis* for patients who are apprehensive or fearful. This appears to be an *unimportant* consideration with respect to premature infants.

"A third consideration is *muscular relaxation*. A child undergoing a resection of bowel, in which there is little or no distention, requires very little, if any, relaxation, whereas one who is

50

being operated upon for omphalocele or diaphragmatic hernia will need maximum relaxation.

"*Obtundation of reflex* activity is a fourth consideration in general anesthesia under certain circumstances. In newborn infants this is probably of *minor importance.*

SUPPORTIVE ROLE

"Maintenance of body warmth should be a major consideration in the care of the premature child undergoing surgery. The infant in the operating room is confronted with air conditioning, use of cold agents for cleansing the skin, use of nonrebreathing circuits in gas machines and use of cold blood for transfusions. All these factors contribute to reduction in body temperature.

"We are becoming increasingly aware of the dangers of using acidified blood for transfusions of infants. If a child faces a major surgical procedure such as removal of a sacrococcygeal teratoma, we believe it is necessary to have fresh blood available and to correct the pH to normal by addition of an alkalinizing medium. Monitoring blood loss is difficult enough with older individuals but it is a critical matter during surgery with small infants."

GUIDE FOR PREOPERATIVE MEDICATION
Before General Anesthesia

AGE	WEIGHT IN KILOGRAMS	WEIGHT IN POUNDS	SCOPOLAMINE OR SCOPOLAMINE	ATROPINE ATROPINE	MORPHINE OR MORPHINE	DEMEROL DEMEROL	NEMBUTAL (SECONAL)
0-6 mo	3-7 kg	7-15 lb	None	0.10 mg	None	None	None
6-12 mo	7-8 kg	15-18 lb	None	0.15 mg	1.0 mg	10 mg	20 mg
12-18 mo	8-11 kg	18-24 lb	0.15 mg	0.2 mg	1.5 mg	15 mg	30 mg
18-24 mo	11-12 kg	24-26 lb	0.15 mg	0.2 mg	2.0 mg	20 mg	35 mg
2-3 yr	12-13 kg	26-29 lb	0.15 mg	0.2 mg	2.5 mg	25 mg	40 mg
3-5 yr	13-18 kg	29-40 lb	0.2 mg	0.3 mg	3 mg	30 mg	55 mg
5-8 yr	18-25 kg	40-55 lb	0.25 mg	0.4 mg	4 mg	40 mg	65 mg
8-10 yr	25-30 kg	55-66 lb	0.3 mg	0.4 mg	5 mg	50 mg	80 mg
10-12 yr	30-36 kg	66-80 lb	None	0.4 mg	6.5 mg	65 mg	100 mg
12-14 yr	36-41 kg	80-90 lb	None	0.5 mg	8 mg	80 mg	120 mg

Chart 13.

Suggested Reading

Smith, Robt. M.: Problems in Anesthetizing a Premature Infant, 49th Ross Conference on Pediatric Research.

ENDOTRACHEAL INTUBATION AND VENTILATION

Some anesthesiologists believe that every child undergoing a major surgical operation should have intratracheal intubation to insure adequate ventilatory support. Others believe that it is quite possible for a small infant who is not distended and who lies in proper position on the operating table to undergo surgery perhaps with local anesthesia and for several hours breathe easily by himself without intubation.

Anesthesiologists agree that endotracheal intubation is indicated in certain circumstances and that it is an atraumtic procedure when performed by those with sufficient experience. If complete relaxation is essential for closure, such as for repair of diaphragmatic hernia or omphalocele or in open chest surgery, the need for controlled ventilation is obvious and mandatory. Re-expansion of collapsed lung tissue after surgery seems to benefit infants and is associated with no particular dangers. This must be done cautiously with minimal positive pressure.

One of the supportive roles of the anesthesiologist consists of monitoring the child. This is particularly difficult with the premature infant about whom it is necessary to determine with some precision cardiac output, peripheral vascular circulation, fluid balance, adequacy of gas exchange and changes in temperature.

LOCAL ANESTHESIA

Local infiltration, used mostly for abdominal procedures, has the advantage of rendering endotracheal intubation unnecessary. It has the disadvantage of not giving the anesthetist good control of the child's airway.

GENERAL ANESTHESIA

Cyclopropane and ether are good general anesthetic agents but have the disadvantage of being explosive, and there are a number of pediatric surgeons who use cautery, even with small children.

Fluothane is a newer agent which many qualified anesthetists believe is not well adapted to use with small children, especially premature infants, because cases of hepatitis have been recognized following use of Fluothane in older patients.

British anesthetists seem to favor the combined use of muscle relaxants and nitrous oxide. It obviously becomes necessary then to perform endotracheal intubation in each child. Of course, with use of relaxants one runs the risk of postoperative respiratory depression. Infants vary considerably in their responses to muscle relaxants, being more susceptible to one type of relaxant and less reactant to another group than are adults.

Most anesthesia in infants is given by way of an Ayre's T-piece. Agents vary but are of secondary importance. A flow of nitrous oxide and oxygen of at least twice the minute volume of the patient is necessary for proper carbon dioxide elimination. This is sometimes supplemented with a low percentage of halothane (0.5% or less) in addition to a muscle relaxant.

It has been shown that in the first six months of life infants are relatively resistant to suxamethonium and sensitive to D-tubo-curarine and that in this respect they resemble patients with myasthenia. Anesthetists usually use suxamethonium intermittently and, in general, avoid the use of D-tubocurarine. In the first few weeks of life, it has been found that the neuro-muscular transmission differs from that in adults in that the block after decamethonium resembles that seen in patients with myasthenia. Aware of this neonatal response to curare, initial doses of 0.25 to 0.5 mg D-tubocurarine, depending on the size of the infant, supplemented with 0.125 gm if necessary, may be used. Neostigmine may be used to reverse the action of D-tubocurarine.

A fall in temperature will aggravate these depressing effects of muscle relaxants. The use of low concentrations of halothane (up to 0.5%) as a supplement to nitrous oxide allows respiration to be controlled with much smaller doses of relaxants than with nitrous oxide alone.

The inter-relationship between pCO_2, pO_2, and cardiac output is related in a linear fashion in that the cardiac output will fall by about 25% when pCO_2 is lowered from 40 to 25 mm Hg. The fall in cardiac output is probably due to decreased catecholamine level. It is prudent, therefore, to mantain the pCO_2 near the normal level.

Blood Replacement: Rapid transfusion of large quantities of cold blood is dangerous and may cause cardiac or total body hypothermia. As heart temperature approaches 30° C there is a great risk of ventricular fibrillation. It is desirable, therefore, to warm the blood prior to transfusion. This may be done either by passing the plastic tube through a warm water bath or by a microwave warmer which is much more rapid and can warm a bag of blood from 5 to 35° C in approximately one minute.

A practical advantage of using prewarmed blood is that it can be transfused about four times as fast. When a large volume of blood is given rapidly calcium should be given to counteract the high potassium content of stored blood.

Humidification: Endotracheal intubation allows for dry gas to reach the lower part of the trachea, by-passing the upper naso-respiratory tract which humidifies, and often allowing for a humidity of only 30% in the inspired gases in the lower tract. This retards ciliary motion. This may increase post-operative problems in that secretions become solidified. It is probable that in the future humidification of anesthetic gases will become more common and certainly this will be desirable.

The infant has a poor respiratory reserve. This is due to a combination of factors: (1) reduction in compliance of the lung may occur due to miliary atelectasis or pulmonary edema, (2) in the premature the respiratory center is easily depressed with anal-gesic drugs, (3) there may be reluctance to cough or breathe deeply due to pain—particularly in thoracic operations. In some instances, if assistance is not given, the patient may become tired due to the increased work-load of breathing which can lead to decreased compliance and rapid deterioration.

The ideal mechanical ventilator has not been designed for the infant. The essentials of an infant ventilator should be (1) the capacity to deliver a tidal volume as low as 15–20 ml (2) enough power to deliver this volume within one second in spite of high resistance and poor lung compliance (3) it must be possible to control the percentage of oxygen (4) good humidification. The Engstrom Respirator probably most nearly fulfills these requirements.

It is relatively easy to humidify air by passing it through a humidifier but as the air passes along the tubing it cools and some condensation occurs. The size of the particle is the major factor that determines the area of the respiratory tract on which the vapour is deposited. Fifty per cent of particles of 1_μ in diameter are deposited in the alveoli and 75–80 per cent of particles more than 4_μ in diameter settle in the upper airway.

Tracheostomy: A tracheostomy may be more safely performed in the infant than was formerly thought if one uses one of the newer silicone type tubes which, when warmed, will adapt to the contour of the trachea. It is also important in avoiding sublaryngeal steno-

to make the incision in the trachea between the second and rd ring and to preserve the first ring. No cartilage should be ised since regeneration does not occur and will result in some ree of narrowing later.

Vhen de-cannulating a child, after tracheostomy, there should be a constant attendant. The child should be sedated to avoid excitement. The sedation used most commonly is 1 mg of morphine sulfate per 10 lb. body weight. If respiratory obstruction appears in spite of sedation, one can assume that there may be an organic obstruction. A bronchoscopy may have to be performed to rule out the possibility of a tracheal granuloma or tracheal flap.

Suggested Reading

Smith, Robert M.: 49th Ross Conf. on Ped. Research.
Wilkinson, A. W.: *Recent Advances in Paediatric Surgery,* Grune & Stratton, Inc., New York, 1969.

Chapter 12

THE NEONATE'S RESPONSE TO
ANTIBIOTICS — USES AND ABUSES

There is often a difference in the neonate's response to antibiotics from that of the adult. Many differences in the infant have to do with dosage. The mycins, particularly Chloromycetin, if given in excessive quantity, may be associated with "gray syndrome" which is characterized by shock, gray appearance, increased salivation, increased tearing and possibly convulsions. Some differences are due to peculiarities in the infant in that some drugs which are not tolerated well by adults are surprisingly well tolerated by the infant. Absorption of a drug may be in an unusual route or at an unusual rate. Conjugation of the drug and/or destruction of the drug may be an unusual process. The infant may excrete the drug in an unusual way or at an unusual rate.

The antibiotics may be classified by their mechanism of effect. The bactericidal antibiotics (Penicillin, Keflin, Vancomycin and Bacitracin) interfere with the synthesis of the bacteria cell wall. The cyclic polypeptides such as Polymyxin, Colistin, Tyrocidine, and Gramicidin disturb the bacteria cell wall and cell membranes. The aminoglycosides such as Streptomycin, Neomycin, Kanamycin, Paromomycin, Gentamicin and Viomycin cause miscoding for the amino acids.

The bacteriostatic antibiotics (Chloromycetin, Tetracyclines, Erythromycin, Lincomycin) interfere with the protein synthesis. Novabiocin which is also bacteriostatic not only interferes with synthesis of protein but also alters the permeability of cell membrane.

The Polyene anti-fungal agents (Amphotericin and Nystatin) interfere with cell membrane permeability.

Optimal therapy of some infections requires the use of more than one antimicrobial agent. In general, combinations of bactericidal agents are synergistic whereas the combination of bactericidal and bacteriostatic drugs tend to decrease the potency.

Before discussing some of the common differences in antibiotics when used in the newborn, it might be noted that attitudes have changed in that where one once felt that a contaminated delivery made it mandatory to treat for potential infection, we now realize that so many of these drugs have special hazards when used in infants, that any advantage of prophylactic antimicrobial drug therapy for the infant with a presumed infection is not so great as previously thought. This is not to say that the infant with obvious serious infection should not receive treatment but certainly an effort should be made to identify the offending bacterial organism and to treat according to the results of the cultures and sensitivities. Enteric organisms are most frequently acquired before or during birth. These include E. Coli and Enteric Streptococci. Post birth infections include commonly the staphylococci, Group B hemolytic streptococci and H. Influenzae. Also after birth one may see aerobacter, paracolon, proteus and pseudomonas organisms contaminating suction machines, bottles and Isolettes. Knowledge of this sequence of the bacterial exposure may prove of some help in the presumed choice of necessary antibacterial agent.

Some of the differences may be outlined as follows:

Penicillin: Some form of penicillin is effective against virtually all of the major infections of the neonate. Penicillin G. is still a very good drug, in addition to being effective against some Gram negative organisms it is also highly effective against most of the Gram positive organisms. Penicillin G is excreted slowly in the premature and in the newborn an aqueous solution in small quantities may sustain therapeutic levels for long periods of time. The use of Procaine may have a damaging effect on urinary excretion. There is an increased incidence of jaundice in the premature given Penicillin G. and Streptomycin and whether the jaundice results from Penicillin G. or Streptomycin or both is not known. In newborn rats, the LD 50 on weight basis was one-seventh of the adult rat LD 50 whether the potassium or sodium salt penicillin was given. For this reason, one should give small doses of aqueous penicillin at only 12 hour intervals. Adequate levels of penicillin are effected by 20,000 U/kg body weight, per dose. Excessive doses of penicillin may cause convulsions. Penicillin G. is still probably the first drug to try in the face of E. Coli infections.

Ampicillin: Ampicillin at 100 mgm/kg body weight/day would be perhaps somewhat superior when faced with a neonatal infection in which the etiological diagnosis has not yet been made.

Kanamycin: Kanamycin (Kantrex) is well tolerated by the neonate and may be added at 15 mg/kg I.M. every 12 hours when the etiology of the infection is unknown. It is a very useful drug in infancy in that the incidence of renal complication is markedly less in comparable doses. Hearing loss in the immature infant is directly related to the dose of kanamycin administered. Infants who have developed deafness have been found to have had excessive doses.

Streptomycin: There is probably very little indication for the use of Streptomycin in the neonate. Many surgeons still give it in combination with Penicillin for peritoneal infections but there are far superior drugs available. Streptomycin, if given for over ten days, may be associated with some eighth nerve changes. This is somewhat related to the dosage. Most individuals will run some albuminuria transiently between the tenth and fourteenth day when on Streptomycin therapy. Excessive doses of Streptomycin to young children produce stupor, flaccidity, coma and respiratory paralysis. This is presumed to be due to interruption of the neuromuscular conduction mechanism. A similar blocking action has been described for both Kanamycin and Neomycin. Deafness with administration of Dihydro-streptomycin is well documented in infants. (McClean *et al.:* reference at back of Chapter 19 in the "Problems of Neonatal Surgery.")

Sulfonamides: McClean and his co-workers found that kernicterus occurred in infants with lower concentrations of bilirubin when concomitantly given sulfonamides. Odell has indicated that not only sulfonamides but salicylates and caffeine sodium benzoate can displace bilirubin from protein to which it is usually bound. This permits bilirubin to infuse into the cells of the brain and thereby produce kernicterus.

Tetracyclines: Tetracyclines are seldom indicated in the newborn. In addition to staining the teeth and causing fluorescence of the bone epiphyses, it frequently may be associated with azotemia and invite super-infections, especially monilia infections. Tetracycline may temporarily slow skeletal growth. This occurs even when the dose is one-fourth the usual therapeutic dose. Tetracyclines in the excessive dosage may also produce "gray syndrome."

They also occasionally cause a febrile condition with associated petechiae with failure of the megakarocites to fragment and be released from the bone marrow. Usual dose 10 mg/Kg/day.

Gentamicin: Gentamicin (Garamycin) is one of the newer effective drugs and is considerably less toxic than Polymyxin and Colistin. It may replace these drugs in the treatment of Pseudomonas infections. It is probably also the drug of choice for Klebsiella infections. A second and third choice for Klebsiella infections would be Cephalothin (Keflin) and Chloramphenicol (Chloromycetin). Gentamicin is also effective against Proteus. Polymycin and Coly-Mycin, due to their renal and neural toxicity, are second choices and are only effective against pseudomonas. While discussing pseudomonas infections, it might be well to mention that 50 percent of the mortality from overwhelming burns are associated with pseudomonas sepsis. This has largely been overcome by the introduction of silver sulfadiazine which, when incorporated into the dressing, makes a painless, effective dressing for 48 hours and is not associated with skin reactions or electrolyte or metabolic disorders as was sulfamyalon. Sulfamyalon is probably no longer indicated in that it causes a marked carbonic anhydrase inhibition and may cause extremely rapid respiration. Usual dose: 4–6 mg/kg/day.

Lincomycin & Erythromycin: These drugs are very similar and are only effective as bacteriostatic agents against gram positive infections. They are of little use in neonatal infections. Although Erythromycin appears to decrease the incidence of neonatal icterus, it apparently is not absorbed and excreted as well by infants as by older children. Usual dose 10 mg/Kg I.M. every 12 hours.

Carbenicillin (Geopen): This is probably the most effective drug that we have for proteus, E. Coli, pseudomonas, and hemophilus infections. It is extremely effective against both gram positive and gram negative organisms; however, it is not effective against Klebsiella. The drawback is that high level doses have to be given and it must be administered either I.M. or I.V. It is excreted in very high concentrations in the urine and has very low toxicity. Occasionally, one may get skin rashes, urticaria, nausea and sometimes phlebitis, as well as thrombocytopenia and granulocytopenia with this drug. Frequently, there is also transient elevation of the SGOT and SGPT. For children, the I.V. Dose for Pseudomonas is

400–500 mg/kg/day in 4 hour interval doses. For Proteus and E. Coli infections this dose may be reduced to 50–200 mg/Kg/day. The drug is stable for 6 hours at room temperature and for 72 hours under refrigeration. It is compatible with virtually all the I.V. fluids on the market.

Keflin: The generic term is Cephalothin and comes from a spore effective against gram negative and gram positive organisms including Penicillinase producing Staph Aureus. Against Pseudomonas, one can reduce the dose of Keflin by two-thirds and the dose of Polymycin by two-thirds and the two have symbiotic action. The average daily dose is 30 mg/pound/day and is given every 4–6 hours I.M. or I.V. There is no accumulative effect. The drug has no toxic effect on the liver or kidneys and is excreted in the urine. It crosses the blood-brain barrier. It is not absorbed in the gastro-intestinal tract but can be given over a long period through an I.V. infusion. It is bactericidal and has a broad spectrum and is also effective against Clostridium, Klebsiella, Aerobacter, Salmonella, Shigella, Paracolon, Hemophilus influenzae, pertussis, Staph Aureus, Strep and pneumonococci. There is no cross resistance and it is unaffected by Penicillin and is rapidly effective in a concentration of 10 Mu/cc in one-half hour after 0.5 gm dose. It is low in toxicity.

Novabiocin: This is a dangerous drug for the neonate. It has been reported to cause a 3-fold increase in the incidence of neonatal icterus. It may be given in doses of 2–4 mg/Kg/day with relative safety but doses in excess of this strikingly increase the chance of icterus.

Bacitracin: Bacitracin is an extremely useful drug in the newborn. The newborn appears to be peculiarly resistant to the toxicity of Bacitracin. It is very important in the administration of this drug that the solution be freshly mixed. Some feel that in unexplained infections of a severe nature that Bacitracin is the drug of choice prior to documentation of the etiology of the infection. This is true only for the newborn age group. Usual dosage 1000 units/kg I.M. every 12 hours (900 units/kg in prematures).

Neomycin and Polymyxin: These drugs have a spectrum similar to Bacitracin but Neomycin must be very carefully used in the peritoneal cavity—absorption may cause neuro-toxicity.

Oxytetracycline (Terramycin): Effective against both gram positive and gram negative organisms. Oral dose is between 10–25 mg/kg/day in 4 doses. I.V. 6 mg/kg/day.

Suggested Reading

Smith, J. W.: *Manual of Medical Therapeutics*, 19th Ed., Little, Brown & Co., Boston, Mass.

Shirkey, H. C.: *Pediatric Therapy*, 4th Ed., C. V. Mosby Co., St. Louis, Mo., 1971.

Charts: *Harriett Lane Handbook.* (Pocket handbook for Johns Hopkins University house staff.)

Barnett, H. L.: *Pediatrics*, 15th Ed., Appleton, Century, Croft, 1972.

Gellis, S. S., and Kagan, B. M.: *Current Pediatric Therapy*, 4th Ed., 1970, p. 762–768, 998.

GUIDE TO THERAPY OF INFECTIONS CAUSED BY SOME COMMON MICROORGANISMS

Antibiotic	Staph. aureus (PCNase negative)	Staph. aureus (PCNase positive)	Str. pyogenes	Viridans strep.	Str. faecalis	Pneumococcus	H. influenzae	Meningococcus	Gonococcus	Kleb. pneumoniae	E. coli	Salmonella	Shigella	Proteus (indole-positive)	Proteus mirabilis (indole-negative)	Pseud. aeruginosa	Aero. aerogenes	M. pneumoniae
Penicillin PCNase-sensitive	+	0	+	+	±	+	±	+	+	0	±	0	0	±	0	0	0	0
Penicillin PCNase-resistant	+	+	+	±	0	+	±	0	0	0	0	0	0	0	0	0	0	0
Ampicillin	+	0	+	+	+	+	+	+	+	±	+	+	+	+	0	0	±	0
Cephalothin	+	+	+	+	0,±	+	±	+	+	+	+	+	+	+	0	0	0	0
Lincomycin	+	+	+	+	0	+	0	0	0	0	0	0	0	0	0	0	0	±
Erythromycin	+	"	+	+	0,±	+	+	+	+	0	0	0	0	0	0	0	0	±
Novobiocin	+	+	±	±	0	+	+	+	+	0	0	0	0	±	±	0	0	?
Vancomycin	+	+	+	+	+	+	0	0	0	0	0	0	0	0	0	0	0	0
Streptomycin	±	*	0	±	±	0	+	0	+	+	+	0	0	±	±	0,±	±	+
Tetracyclines	+	*	±	0	0	+	+	+	+	+	+	0	±	0,±	±	0	±	+
Chloramphenicol	+	*	0,±	0	0	+	+	+	+	+	+	+	+	+	±	0	±	+
Kanamycin	+	+	0	0	0	0	0	+	+	+	+	±	+	±	+	0	+	±
Polymyxin B, colistin	0	0	0	0	0	0	+	0	0	+	+	+	+	0	0	+	+	0
Cephaloridine	+	+	+	+	0,±	+	±	+	+	+	+	+	+	+	0	0	0	0
Sulfonamides	0	0	±	0	0	+	+	+	±	±	±	0	±	±	±	0	±	?
Nitrofurantoin†	0	0	+	0	±	±	0	0	0	±	±	0	0	±	±	0	±	?
Nalidixic acid†	0	0	0	0	0	0	±	+	+	+	+	+	+	+	±	0	+	?

A plus (+) indicates that the organism is usually sensitive to the antibiotic; + indicates variable sensitivity; and 0 indicates unlikely sensitivity (or resistance). Gray circle indicates the preferred antimicrobials for each species of infecting organism.

This table is intended only as a guide to the activities of certain antibiotics; selection of the appropriate antimicrobial depends on the clinical circumstances and the antibiotic sensitivity tests. For therapeutic effectiveness, the minimal inhibitory concentration (MIC) of the antibiotic for any specific organism (as determined in a tube-dilution sensitivity test) should be at least 4–8 times less than an achievable serum concentration. Dilutions of the patient's serum may be tested directly against the organism as a check on the serum antimicrobial activity.

* Penicillinase is not active against these drugs, but organisms that have been induced to produce penicillinase often have been exposed to these antibiotics and have developed resistance.

† Serum levels are very low; useful only in urinary tract infections. Resistance may develop rapidly to nalidixic acid.

Chart 14. Guide to therapy of infections.

RELATION OF ANTIBIOTIC DOSAGE TO SERUM CONSENTRATION

| Antibiotic | Route of Administration and Dose | | | Serum Concentration† |
	Intravenous	Intramuscular	Oral	
Crystalline PCN G	1-5 (million) units every 4-6 hrs	-	-	4
Procaine PCN G	-	0.3-1.2 M units every 6-12 hrs	-	2-3
Phenoxymethyl PCN, phenethicillin	-	-	0.25-1 gm every 6 hrs	0.1-2.0
Benzathine PCN	-	1.2 units every 2-4 wks	-	0.01-0.1
Methicillin	1-2 gm every 4-6 hrs	1-2 gm every 4-6 hrs	-	6-10
Oxacillin	0.5-1 gm every 4-6 hrs	0.5-1gm every 4-6 hrs	0.25-1 gm every 4-6 hrs	4-13
Cloxacillin	0.5-1 gm every 4-6 hrs	0.25-0.5 gm every 6 hrs	0.25-1 gm every 4-6 hrs	6-10
Dicloxacillin	0.5-1 gm every 4-6 hrs	0.25-0.5 gm every 4-6 hrs	0.25-0.5 gm every 4-6 hrs	10
Nafcillin	1-2 gm every 4-6 hrs	0.5 gm every 4-6 hrs	0.25-1 gm every 4-6 hrs	5-8
Ampicillin	0.5 gm every 6 hrs	0.5-1 gm every 6 hrs	0.25-1 gm every 6 hrs	2-8
Cephalothin	1-2 gm every 4-6 hrs	1 gm every 4-6 hrs	-	20
Cephaloridine	0.25-1.0 gm every 6 hrs	0.25-1.0 gm every 6 hrs	-	10-35
Lincomycin	0.6 gm every 8-12 hrs	0.6 gm every 12 hrs	0.5 gm every 6-8 hrs	2-20
Erythromycin	0.5-1 gm every 6 hrs	0.2 gm every 4-6 hrs	0.25-1 g every 6 hrs	0.5-10
Oleandomycin	0.2-0.4 gm every 6 hrs	0.2-0.4 gm every 6 hrs	0.25-0.5 gm every 6 hrs‡	1-10
Novobiocin	0.25-0.5 gm every 6 hrs	0.25-0.5 gm every 6 hrs	0.25-0.5 gm every 6 hrs	10-30
Vancomycin	0.5 gm every 6 hrs	-	-	6-25
Streptomycin	1-2 gm daily	0.5-1 gm every 12 hrs	-	20-30
Tetracyclines	0.25 gm every 6 hrs (not over 1 gm/day)	-	0.25-0.5 gm every 6 hrs (0.15 gm every 6 hrs for demethylchortetra-cycline)	3-5
Chloramphenicol	0.5-1 gm every 6 hrs	0.5-1 gm every 6 hrs	0.25-1 gm every 6 hrs	10-20
Kanamycin	15 mg/kg/day in 2 doses (not over 1.5 gm/day)	15 mg/kg/day in 2 doses (not over 1.5 gm/day)	-	2-30
Polymyxin B	2.5 mg/kg/day in 4 doses	1.5-2.5 mg/kg day in 4 doses	-	1-8
Colistin		2.5-5 mg/kg/day in 2-4 doses	-	3-5

† Serum concentrations are approximations of those achieved with the lower dosage schedules and are expressed in units/ml for crystalline, procaine, and benzathine PCN, and in µg/ml for all other drugs.
‡ Triacetyl derivative.

Chart 15. These doses relate to the adult doses that should be compared with the square meter body surface charts for interpretation to the infant or child.

ANTIBIOTICS IN UREMIA

ANTIBIOTIC	SERUM HALF-LIFE (In Hours)		ALSO REMOVED BY	DOSE MODIFICATION	MODIFIED DOSE INTERVAL (In Hours) in AZOTEMIA	
	NORMAL	OLIGURIA			Clcr 10	Clcr 10
Cephalothin	0.5-0.8	3-18	Liver	Minor	24	12
Chloramphenicol	1.6-3.3	3-4	Liver	None		
Chlortetracycline	5.6	7-11	Liver	Do Not Use		
Colistin	2	48-72	?	Major	72-96	36-48
Erythromycin	1.4	5-6	Liver	None		
Kanamycin	3	72-96	?	Major	72-96	36-48
Methicillin	0.5	4	Liver	None		
Oxacillin	0.5	2	Marked	None		
Penicillin G	0.5	7-10	Liver	Minor	8-10	4-5
Polymyxin B	6	48-72	?	Major	72-96	36-48
Streptomycin	2.5	52-100	?	Major	72-96	36-48
Tetracycline	8.5	57-108	Liver	Major	72-96	36-48

DOSAGES OF ANTIBIOTICS IN UREMIA

Modifications are based primarily on serum half-lives of the antibiotics in anuric patients.

A single dose of the antibiotic is given based on a q6h, q8h or q12h schedule, but all subsequent doses are halved and given at intervals based on the following table. For example: If a child were to normally receive 10 mg/kg/day of Kanamycin as 5 mg/kg q12h, then he would get 5 mg/kg initially but the interval before the next dose of 2.5 mg/kg would be 36-48 hours (Clcr 10 ml/minute) or 72-96 hours (Clcr 10 ml/minute) later.

Extreme caution must be exercised and these dosage modifications are approximations only. Serum levels of antibiotics at appropriate intervals should be measured and dosage and/or interval adjusted according to serum levels and early signs of toxicity.

Chart 16. Antibiotics in uremia.

Chapter 13

BURNS

The mortality and morbidity associated with major burns in infants and children is considerably higher than that seen in adults and older children. This may be due in part to the common practice of using the Brooke Army Hospital formula which dangerously overloads the circulation of the infant.

In estimating body surface burned, instead of using the conventional "rule of 18"; in the infant one should use a "rule of 13" in that the head and neck surface area consititutes 13% in the infant (rather than 9% as in the adult); both upper extremities combine to constitute 13% (versus 18% in the adult); each leg is 13% (18% in adult); the remaining 48% is equally divided between the front and back of the torso.

As a useful "rule of thumb" to anticipate the complications and causes of death according to the chronological sequence in acute burns, one may use a "rule of sevens" which has been devised by this author:

(1) The first 7 *hrs.* the chief cause of death will be *asphyxiation*.
(2) At 72 *hrs.* a second cause of death will be due to *unremitting shock*.
(3) At 7 *days* a third cause of death will be *renal shut-down with potassium intoxication*.
(4) At 7 *weeks* a fourth cause of death will be due to *infection* usually associated with gram-negative sepsis.

Two relatively new drugs, Sulfamyalon and Garamycin, have greatly altered this last cause of death in that they reduce the total bulk of gram-negative organisms per square centimeter of burned flesh in a remarkable way.

SKIN SURFACE AREA ADULT

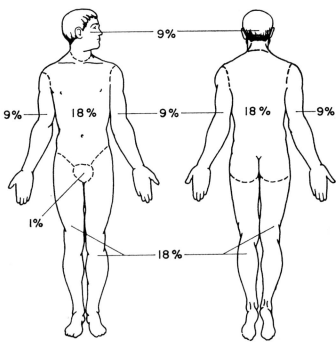

Chart 17. This represents the comparison of surface areas for estimation of the percentage of burns as seen in the adult and older child versus the infant.

For purposes of illustration, one may take the sequence of management that would apply to a typical 40% third degree burn involving the face and associated with circumferential burns of the knees and thighs. The three first areas of concern would be:

(1) Inhalation of flames with imminent possibility of asphyxiation.
(2) Shock due to acute fluid loss into the burn.
(3) Potential renal shut-down associated with shock and possible condensation of acid hematin crystals in the kidney.

After evaluating the respiratory situation, it is determined that this child has a fair amount of laryngeal stridor and in order to properly control the respiratory toilet a tracheotomy is performed. Since there are burns on the upper chest and neck region which preclude a transsubclavian vein catheter, after appropriately prepping the groin area, a silicone catheter is placed through the

SKIN SURFACE AREA INFANT

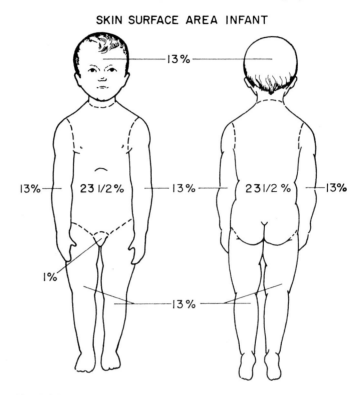

Chart 18. This represents the comparison of surface areas for estimation of the percentage of burns as seen in the adult and older child versus the infant.

saphenous bulb into the inferior vena cava. This area has been meticulously cleaned and a very firm occlusive dressing placed over this cutdown area since this will be the major "life-line" for the patient's nutrition over the ensuing weeks. Next, the consideration of shock and renal shut-down is discussed with the house staff as well as the proper precautions to maintain a sterile environment as far as possible. Colloid of either plasma or whole blood, with 1 cc per percent burn/kg body wgt. is started. This will be given over the first 24 hrs. together with 2 cc/kg of a solution containing 5% dextrose in saline with 2% urea. This will usually allow for the urinary flow to be maintained in an infant under lyr. at 15 cc/hr. and in older children at 20 cc/hr. The urine will, at first, be somewhat pink but will rapidly clear. The rate of fluid injection will be ½ of the colloid dose for 24 hrs.

given in the first 8 hrs. and remaining dose over the next 16 hrs. Similarly, $1/2$ of the other I.V. fluids are given in the first 8 hrs. and remaining spread over the next 16 hrs. The non-colloid fluid, however, may be adjusted so as to maintain urinary flow: in this particular patient (infant), 15–20 cc/hr. Urinary flow will largely determine the rate of major fluid administration.

The infant is placed on sterile sheets; cap and gown with pHisohex scrub technique instituted for all those coming into contact with the patient. The patient is isolated and allowed only supervised visiting to allay fear.

Once control of the respiratory tract is established and suction routine instituted including the use of a tracheotomy tube of silicone and use of urea to maintain an hourly urinary output, an intake-output chart is begun which records at two hour intervals the gross intake and output which is totaled on an eight hour basis. A thin layer of Garamycin ointment is placed over the burned area and this is repeated every 12 hrs. Sterile sheets are changed every 12 hrs. In the infant, the lower extremities are covered with Furacin pressure occlusive dressings to cut down on fecal contamination. Once the patient is stabilized from the standpoint of respiration and circulatory blood volume and adequate urinary output is assured, plans are then made to try to prevent contractures around the knee where some of the tendons are rather superficial. An operative program which envisions the use of very light anesthetic or Ketamine is planned to remove the third degree circumferential burn around the knee and to graft immediately to insure early function and also to cut the percentage of third degree burn from 40% down to 30% area. The graft donor site in this case would be the back—long strips of skin are taken and wrapped in an oblique fashion about the debrided knees. A pressure occlusive dressing is applied after first overlying the grafts with Furacin strips. Dressings are changed every 4 days and graft "take" under these circumstances should be 100%. After function is assured about joints involved, cosmetic considerations of the bulk areas which may lead to gram negative sepsis become the next areas of attention.

Drugs which are very useful in topical application for severe burns and which greatly reduce the bacteria per sq. centimeter of burned tissue are Sulfamylon and Garamycin.

Suggested Reading

Metcoff, J., *et al.:* Requirements for Water and Electrolytes after Extensive Burns, *New England J Med, 265*:101, 1961.

Mecker, I. A.: Dermatone Debridement, Early Grafting and Management of Extensive Burns in Children, *Ped, 29*:865, 1962.

Polk, H. C., and Stone, H. H.: *Contemporary Burn Management,* Little, Brown and Co., 1971.

Chapter 14

CANCER IN CHILDHOOD

Tumor therapy has been greatly benefited by the work at St. Jude's Hospital in Memphis, Tennessee. The subject of tumor therapy is a very dynamic one, undergoing constant change. The following comments relate to St. Jude's format for tumor therapy and one can gain much from reviewing the thinking of one of their leading investigators, Dr. David H. James, Jr.

"Cancer, in the United States, is second only to accidents as a cause of death between the ages of 1 and 14 years and accounts for approximately 20 percent of deaths from disease during this period of life. Despite improvements in surgical techniques, radiotherapy, chemotherapy and general supportive care, the death rate from childhood cancer has remained essentially unchanged during recent years."

Unfortunately, the majority of children with malignant tumors have local or distant metastases at the time of the original diagnosis. It is, therefore, frequently impossible to accomplish complete eradication of the malignancy by surgical excision alone. However, much palliation, and occasionally complete eradication, can be accomplished by the optimal use of radiation therapy and chemotherapy in addition to the surgical procedures. Therefore, it is essential that there be close coordination between the surgeon, radiotherapist, pathologist and cancer chemotherapist if the best possible results are to be obtained.

The most common types of cancer in childhood are leukemia, brain tumors, neuroblastoma, Wilm's tumor, rhabdomyosarcoma, lymphomas and bone tumors.

NEUROBLASTOMA

Excluding brain tumors, neuroblastoma is the most common

type of malignant solid tumor of childhood. It is thought to be derived from the primitive sympathetic neuroblast of neural crest origin. Histologically, it may consist entirely of undifferentiated small round cells or may be a mixture of undifferentiated neuroblasts, and mature ganglion cells. The amount of pleomorphism varies from case to case. In general, the degree of malignancy of a particular tumor is inversely related to the percentage of ganglion cells present. "Rosettes" are a characteristic histological feature of this tumor but are not seen in every case.

Approximately 50–60% of neuroblastomas have their clinical onset during the first four years of life; however, they can become manifest at any age during childhood. The most common site of the primary tumor is the retroperitoneal space in the upper part of the abdomen; either in the adrenal medulla or in one of the adjacent sympathetic ganglia. The primary tumor may also arise in sympathetic ganglia of the neck, thorax, lower abdomen or pelvis. At times there appear to be multiple sites of origin and occasionally no primary site can be found.

The clinical signs and symptoms of neuroblastoma may appear suddenly or they may have an insidious onset. Most often the early manifestations are of nonspecific nature, such as anorexia, weight loss, fever, listlessness, pallor, anemia and bone or joint pain. Unfortunately, local or distant metastases are usually present at the time a palpable primary tumor is first noted.

Late findings may include periorbital swelling and hemorrhages, proptosis, subconjunctival hemorrhages, lymphadenopathy, separation of cranial sutures, swelling and tenderness of bones and joints, severe anemia, thrombocytopenia, and signs and symptoms of pressure on the brain, spinal cord, airway, rectum and/or bladder.

Roentgenographic studies are usually very helpful in the diagnostic evaluation. An intravenous pyelogram may show displacement of the kidney or ureter without much distortion of the renal pelvis or calyceal system. Calcification may be seen in the suprarenal area or, more rarely, in the lower part of the abdomen. A chest x-ray may demonstrate the presence of a mass in the posterior mediastinum which may or may not be producing symptoms. The long bones may appear "moth-eaten" or "mottled" and there may be signs of periosteal reaction. Occasionally, a pathologic fracture is observed. The cranial sutures may be separated and osteolytic lesions may be seen in the skull, vertebrae, ribs, pelvis, clavicle or scapula. In those instances in which the tumor has extended through an intervertebral foramina, a myelogram may reveal partial obliteration of the subarachnoid space.

Children with neuroblastoma frequently have tumor cells in the bone marrow at the time of the original diagnosis. These may appear as individual cells, rosettes, clumps of cells or there may be complete replacement of all the normal marrow elements. The presence of neuroblasts in the marrow can help establish the diagnosis in some cases and be of aid in planning treatment.

The urinary excretion of the catecholamines or their breakdown products is frequently elevated in children with neuroblastoma. In many clinics the vanilmandelic acid (VMA) and homovanillic acid (HVA) determinations have been the most helpful, both for diagnosis and as an aid in following response to treatment.

Neuroblastoma grows well in tissue culture and has a characteristic morphological appearance. This procedure can be of value at times in helping to establish a definitive diagnosis.

The treatment of neuroblastoma depends upon the extent of disease at the time of the diagnosis. In those rare instances in which the tumor is well-localized and encapsulated, surgical excision should be done as soon as is practical. Postoperative radiation therapy to the tumor bed is administered in most clinics. However, decisions concerning radiation should be individualized.

If the tumor is localized or regional, but unresectable, two approaches are possible. Either an attempt should be made to reduce the size by the use of radiation therapy or chemotherapy, or a combination of these two modalities in order that the tumor can be completely resected, or as much of the tumor should be excised as possible and the residual tumor should then be treated with radiation alone or radiation plus chemotherapy.

In patients with generalized neuroblastoma, the treatment of choice is chemotherapy. The most effective drugs at the present time are the alkylating agent, cyclophosphamide, and the alkaloid, vincristine sulfate. In some patients, much palliation can be achieved with these agents and an occasional long-term survival can be obtained.

Supportive treatment with blood transfusions, analgesics and radiation therapy to control bone pain is important in the overall management of the child.

DIAGNOSIS OF NEUROBLASTOMA

VMA has become a common household word in hospital jargon. Many investigators have reported increased urinary excretion of the products of catacholamines. Foremost among these are Voorhees and Gardner, Von Studnitz, and Kaser *et al.*, who have described the increased urinary excretion of 3-methoxy-4 hydroxymandelic acid (VMA) and homovanillic acid (HVA) that occurs in patients with neuroblastoma. In spite of these reports, biochemical studies of the urine from patients in which neuroblastoma is suspected have not yet become commonplace. Even though not all patients with neuroblastoma show the elevated urinary excretion of VMA, HVA, and other metabolites of norepinephrine and its precursors, marked elevations are present in about 75% of these patients. This paper describes a very simple test which may be applied to the urine of patients suspected of having neuroblastoma, or in whom neuroblastoma should be considered in the differential diagnosis. This test is based on the reaction of dilute diazotized para-nitroaniline with the phenolic metabolites of norepinephrine and its precursors in a spot of urine from the patient.

MATERIALS AND METHODS

Reagents

(1) 0.2% p-nitroaniline,
(2) 0.2% sodium nitrite solution,
(3) 10% potassium carbonate.

The p-nitroaniline solution is prepared by dissolving 1 gm of p-nitroaniline in 10 ml of concentrated HC 1, the solution is then diluted up to 500 ml with distilled water. The sodium nitrite solution is prepared by dissolving 1 gm of $NaNO_2$ in 500 ml of distilled water. The 10% potassium carbonate solution is prepared by dissolving 50 gm of K_2CO_3 in distilled water and diluting up to 500 ml. These solutions are stored in the refrigerator at 4° C and then are immediately ready for preparation of the spray reagent.

The spray reagent is prepared by mixing equal volumes of the p-nitroaniline and cold sodium nitrite solutions; the yellow color of the p-nitroaniline should turn almost colorless after these two reagents are mixed. This color change is almost instantaneous. The resulting solution is mixed with an equal volume of the 10% potassium carbonate solution and the alkaline reagent is used *within 2 minutes.*

One drop of the urine specimen to be tested is placed on a piece of filter paper allowed to dry; it is then sprayed with alkaline diazotized paranitroaniline which is prepared as described above.

Urine specimens from patients with neuroblastoma and other neural crest tumors turn a strong purple color which is due to VMA. A blue halo which is occasionally present is due to homovanillic acid. Normal urine specimens show a yellow central area with a faint purple perimeter. For comparison, it is advisable to run a urine specimen from a normal person at the same time as the one from the patient suspected of having a neural crest tumor.

When the spot test is positive, it is desirable to check two urine specimens at least 24 hours apart before further study. In *all* urine specimens which give positive reactions, it is essential to identify the compounds which are producing the colored product. One single procedure by which this identification may be accomplished is to acidify the urine, extract with ethyl acetate, concentrate the ethyl acetate and prepare two-dimensional chromatograms as described by Armstrong, Shaw and Wall.

RESULTS

Compounds of dietary origin or metabolites of drugs such as vanillic acid, guaiacol, Darvon, etc., frequently give positive spot tests, but are easily identified by their characteristic migration on the two-dimensional chromatograms. The compound which is most difficult to differentiate from VMA is 3-methoxy-4-hydroxy-phenylhydracrylic acid (MHPHA). However, MHPHA is broken down by heating acidified urine to 100° C for one hour, whereas VMA is quite stable under these conditions.

Positive spot tests have been found in 12 of 16 (75%) patients with histologically proven neural crest tumors, and in only 15% of pediatric patients without neural crest tumors and *not* on dietary control. The nature of the reactive material was identified by two-dimensional chromatography in the latter group of patients.

The simplicity of this test strongly encourages its use in examination of the patients in whom neuroblastoma should be considered.

TUMOR DIAGNOSIS AND THERAPY

Tumor diagnosis and therapy are two of the most important aspects of nonoperative pediatric surgery. An up-to-date protocol for tumor therapy is often hard to come by since it is a dynamic subject and constantly changing. Cancer, second only to accidents as the chief cause of death in ages one to fourteen, should be an important subject to all those who care for children. Only leukemia and central nervous system tumors have a higher incidence than solid tumors in childhood. Approximately 20% of the deaths in ages one to fourteen are due to some malignant, solid tumor.

As mentioned previously, the most common types of cancer in children are leukemia, brain tumors, neuroblastoma, Wilm's tumor, rhabdomyosarcoma, lymphomas and bone tumors. Leukemia, brain tumors and bone tumors will be excluded from this discussion.

Neuroblastoma

Neuroblastoma, next to brain tumors, is the most common type of malignant, solid tumor in childhood. It may occur anywhere along the primitive Islands of Zuckercandle from the cervical sympathetic chain to the pelvic sympathetic chain. Microscopically, it consists of a mixture of undifferentiated neuroblasts and ganglion cells. It may be called a neuroblastoma, or a ganglioneuroblastoma; depending on the relationship of the number of ganglion cells to the other cells. Undifferentiated small, round cells are frequently seen throughout the tumor. One may say that the degree of malignancy appears to be related to the percentage of ganglion cells. The more ganglion cells present the less malignant the tumor.

Like Wilm's tumor, neuroblastoma survival and/or cure is

directly related to age of onset. In general, the survival rate is much higher if the diagnosis is made in the first year of life and therapy instituted. Both neuroblastoma and Wilm's tumor have suggestive evidence that they are congenital in origin in that tumor masses have been found in fetuses. Neuroblastoma may appear to have a sudden onset—most frequently due to hemorrhage into the tumor. The most common presenting sign is that the mother feels a mass while bathing the child. The child may also have some fever, be listless and pale. While local or distal metastasis may frequently be present at the time the tumor is discovered, unless there is x-ray evidence of metastasis to the bones, the prognosis is unpredictable and may be quite good.

There are many fascinating aspects of neuroblastoma—it may be cultured and will grow dendrites. Seventy-five percent of the patients with neuroblastoma have an elevated urinary excretion of VMA, HVA or other metabolities of norepinephrine and its precursors. A sudden increase in tumor growth is apparently due to a sudden increase in tumor circulation. Dr. Judah Folkman has demonstrated that the tumor, when in a very small stage, may have a factor which calls forth a centripital increase in blood vessel alignment towards the small tumor—and that once the tumor receives its own contiguous blood supply by contact of these vessels with the tumor, the tumor may blossom forth very rapidly. (See last chapter.)

Dr. Alexander Bill and associates in Seattle have made some very interesting observations. In 500 autopsies of newborns, they found a forty times increase in expectancy of the incidence of neuroblastoma. This suggested the possibility that neuroblastoma may actually be present and undergo a spontaneous "cure" much more often than we recognize. There have been 28 proven cases of spontaneous regression of neuroblastoma. Dr. Bill and his associates have also developed a tumor growth substance which can be assayed. This substance, when given to the tumor in experimental animals, will cause tremendous overgrowth of the various ganglion and nerve substances. They have also developed an antitumor substance which will cause regression of the tumor.

Diagnostically, one should get norepinephrine output, homovanillic acid output, and VMA output in the urine. The chance of having a positive VMA in some studies run 35–75%; whereas the combined diagnostic tests jump to positive in over 80% if all three tests are done. Associated with the increased output of nore-pinephrine products, the patient may have side symptoms of asthma and/or a pseudo-celiac type of picture. These signs and symptoms regress with complete resection of the tumor. A some-what similar tumor in origin is the carcinoid tumor which also is associated with an increased output of norepinephrine prod-ucts but which has the peripheral symptoms only when there is liver metastasis. Neuroblastoma is apparently able to have in-creased output of norepinephrine products un-associated with liver metastasis.

A simple laboratory test designed by Dr. Elwood H. LaBrosse may be useful as a screening test for some of these peripheral metabolites in suspected cases of neuroblastoma. This test is based on the reaction of dilute diazotized paranitroaniline with phenolic metabolites of norepinephrine and its precursors in a spot of urine from the patient. A color change is almost instan-taneous when any of these metabolites are present. One drop of the urine specimen to be tested is placed on a piece of filter paper and allowed to dry; it is then sprayed with alkaline diazotized paranitroaniline. Urine specimens from patients with neuroblas-toma and other neural crest tumors turn a strong purple color which is due to VMA. A blue halo which is occasionally present is due to HVA. A new "diaper test" or dipstick determination of VMA in the urine of infants has been developed.

The ultimate outlook for the treatment of neuroblastoma is so unpredictable that one should be prepared to take certain chances in the hope for an effective cure. Dr. C. Everett Koop has dem-onstrated that just macerating the tumor or removing part of it is associated with a 38% cure rate. A combination of chemother-apy may make a formerly unresectable tumor resectable.

The current use of the antibiotic, Dactinomycin, and the alka-loid Vincrystine Sulfate, have produced tumor regression in chil-dren with a number af malignant neoplasms, namely neuroblas-toma, Wilm's tumor, and rhabdomyosarcoma. The anti-tumor spectrum of Vincrystine Sulfate includes lymphomas, Wilm's tumors, rhabdomyosarcomas, neuroblastomas, Ewing's tumor, ret-inoblastomas and lyposarcomas. Dactinomycin acts by binding the guanane moiety of deoxyribonucleic acid and thereby prevents the formation of ribonucleic acid polymerase. As a result, ribo-nucleic acid and protein synthesis are suppressed and cellular damage occurs. Although the specific mechanism of the action of Vincrystine Sulfate is unknown, it apparently prevents cell division by interfering with the formation of the spindle tubules of the mitotic apparatus. The limiting factor of Dactinomycin is bone marrow depression and the limiting factor of Vincrystine Sulfate is neurotoxicity. Since both drugs have been shown to cause regression in a small percentage of cases of neuroblastoma, the combined and additive anti-tumor effect has been tried very successfully. Apparently, the toxic effects are not additive.

Vincrystine Sulfate and Cyclophosphamide were administered concurrently to 9 consecutive children with unresectable neuroblastomas at St. Jude's Hospital by Dr. David James and his associates. All 9 children had objective tumor regression and there was complete regression in 7 patients. Findings of this report indicate that the concurrent use of Vincrystine Sulfate and Cyclophosphamide produce prolonged, symptom-free survival of children with neuroblastoma. Some unresectable neuroblastomas will respond to chemotherapy alone and when followed by x-ray therapy may allow for complete surgical excision.

Dactinomycin is dissolved 1 mgm to 4 cc of water and is administered immediately after mixing. The total dose is 2.5 mgm/sq meter body surface, I.V., in 4 divided doses over 8–14 days. Vincrystine Sulfate is mixed 1 mgm to 2 cc of saline given immediately. This should be given concurrently with Dactinomycin. The Vincrystine Sulfate mixture is administered I.V. for 5–6 weeks in single weekly doses of 1.5 mgm/sq meter body surface area. The addition of 2500 R radiation therapy may further reduce the residual tumor; thereby increasing the chance of making a so-called inoperable tumor operable. One of the best examples of concurrent use of chemotherapeutic agents for treatment of a single disease is that of Streptomycin with izoniazid in the treatment of tuberculosis. With lymphatic leukemia the use of Mercaptopurine and Methotrexate concurrently is more effective in producing remissions. In malignant testicular tumor the use of Chlorambucil, Dactinomycin and Methotrexate appears to be most effective. Cyclophosphamed and Vincrystine Sulfate are logical choices of drug treatment in childhood neuroblastoma. Each has a therapeutic effect against neuroblastoma and has a different mechanism of action. The toxic effects are different and do not appear to be additive. Therefore, additive therapeutic effects can be achieved without additive toxic effects.

Suggested Reading

Voorhess, M. L., and Gardner, L. I.: Catecholamine Metabolism in Neuroblastomas, *Lancet, II*:651, 1960.

Von Studnitz, W.: Über die Asscheidung der 3 Methoxy-4-Hydrox-phenylessigsäure (Homovanillinsäure) bein Neuroblastom und anderen neurolen tumoren. *Klin Wschr, 40*:163, 1962.

Käser, Von H., Schweisguth, O., Sellei, K., and Spengler, G. A.: Die Klinische Bedeutung der Bestimmung von Katechinaminkata-boliten bein Tumoren, *Helvetica Medica Acta, 30*:628, 1963.

Armstrong, M. D., McMillan, A., and Shaw, K. N. F.: 3-Methoxy-4-hydroxy-DOMandelic Acid, A Urinary Metabolite of Norepine-phrine, *Biochem Biophys Acta, 25*:422, 1957.

Acheson, R. M., Paul, R. M., and Tomlinson, R. V.: Some Constitu-ents of the Urine of Normal and Schizophrenic Individuals. *Can J Biochem Physiol, 36*:295, 1958.

Armstrong, M. D., Shaw, K. N. F. and Wall, P. E.: The Phenolic Acids of Human Urine: Paper Chromatography of Phenolic Acids. *J Biol Chem, 218*:293, 1956.

SOME RECENT THOUGHTS CONCERNING NEUROBLASTOMA

The subject of neuroblastoma has many parameters. It is one of the most dynamic subjects in tumor therapy. The most excit-ing work on this subject has come from Seattle by Dr. Alexander Bill and his associates. Some of their findings are summarized in the following paragraphs.

"There is a remarkable difference between the types of tumors seen in children and those seen in adults. While carcinoma com-prises 90% of malignant tumors seen in adult life, it comprises only 4% of the malignancies of infancy and childhood. Most of the other malignant tumors of infants and children are unique to this age group.

"Evidence for immune mechanisms in neuroblastoma patients against the tumor include:

"(1) The finding of infiltrates of lymphocytes in the tumors from patients having a good prognosis;

"(2) In tissue culture, there appears to be a lethal immune reaction by the lymphocytes of neuroblastoma patients against the tumor cells;

"(3) A less constant lethal immune activity by the plasma against tumor cells in tissue culture; and

"(4) Unfavorable immune factor has been demonstrated which is a humoral "blocking antibody."

"Among infants in the first year of life, there is a correlation between higher blood lymphocyte counts at diagnosis and survival, and between lower counts and nonsurvival.

"Lymphocytes from four of five mothers whose children had neuroblastomas inhibited tumor cells from the mother's own children and from other children to the same extent. Plasma from some neuroblastoma patients and from some mothers of neuroblastoma patients decreased the plating efficiency of neuroblastoma cells if active complement was supplied."

A brief review of the information that has been accumulated during the past three years in Seattle and elsewhere concerning neuroblastoma is in order.

(1) It has been demonstrated by the collective review of Everson and Cole that babies with neuroblastoma apparently have the highest rate of spontaneous regression of any type of malignancy which afflicts man. While this is only of the order of 5 to 10 percent, it is significant.

(2) Review of their series of cases and of the material in our own hospital has demonstrated the fact that most of these children get better (if they are going to) by disappearance of the tumor cells, rather than by maturation, as had previously been thought. Certainly a few tumors become benign by maturation, but most cures are by tumor-cell disappearance.

(3) The work of Beckwith and Perrin on autopsy studies of infants who died of other diseases has shown that neuroblastomas are present in routine autopsies of infants up to the age of 3 months at 40 times the clinically expected rate of appearance. They did not see these so-called *in situ* neuroblastomas after the age of 3 months. This means that for every 100 clinical cases seen there were presumably 4,000 tumors in newborn infants which then spontaneously disappeared without making their appearance as clinical disease.

(4) They have made exhaustive studies of the possibility of a

relationship between the nerve factor of Levi-Montalcini and the behavior of neuroblastoma. These studies have shown no convincing correlation between the two.

(5) Studies of their pathology specimens of neuroblastoma were carried out in the pathology department by Drs. Martin and Beckwith. They examined these specimens for infiltrates with plasma cells and lymphocytes. They demonstrated that such infiltrates could be seen in cases which were proven to have a good prognosis. This has been regarded in other tumors as evidence of an immune reaction, and could be so regarded in this tumor.

(6) Starting a little over a year ago, they have had the privilege of the collaboration of Drs. Ingegerd and Karl Erik Hellstrom and Dr. George Pierce, working at the University of Washington School of Medicine, in a search for immune reactions to this tumor. These have been found, as has been reported elsewhere.

This discovery should be put in perspective with the rest of the cancer problem. This is the third human malignancy in which immune reactions have been demonstrated *in vitro*. The first two were Burkitt's tumor and melanoma. In these two tumors, an immune reaction could be demonstrated by the immune fluorescence test, which demonstrated a reaction between the patient's serum and tumor cells. This test simply shows the presence of an immune reaction. It says nothing about whether this reaction is lethal to the cells or not. With the colony inhibition test of Ingegerd Hellstrom, immune reactions have been demonstrated for the first time in a human tumor by the lymphocytes, as well as by the plasma. In addition to this, the test demonstrates that these immune reactions are lethal to the cells in tissue culture. Therefore, what has been demonstrated is widely regarded as a milestone of great significance in the study of the biology of malignancy.

Suggested Reading

Bill, Alexander: The Implications of Immune Reactions to Neuro-
    blastoma, *Surgery,* *66*:415–418, No. 2, Aug. 69.
Bill, Alexander, and Morgan, Allen: Evidence of Immune Reaction
    to Neuroblastoma and Future Possibilities for Investigation, *J
    Ped Surg,* *5*: No. 2, April 1970.
Bill, Alexander, *et al.*: Unique Biology of Childhood Tumors, *Pacific
    Med & Surg,* *75*:281–284, Sep-Oct, 67.

RETINOBLASTOMA

Retinoblastoma, a malignant tumor of the eye, is related closely, both histologically and biologically, to neuroblastoma. Although much less common than neuroblastoma it is important to keep in mind because the prognosis is good if the diagnosis is made early.

The earliest sign of retinoblastoma is usually an opacity behind the pupil in an infant or small child. This opacity may be white, grey, yellow or a mixture of these colors. Strabismus and a dilated pupil are frequently present. A careful examination by an opthalmologist will usually establish the diagnosis. However, the tumor should be suspected by the physician who is following the infant and supervising the well-baby care.

If the tumor is limited to the globe of one eye, treatment consists of simple enucleation of the involved eye. However, if there has been extension of the tumor along the optic nerve or into the tissues of the orbit, radiation and chemotherapy should be administered following the enucleation. In those instances in which the tumor is bilateral, the eye with the most far-advanced tumor should be enucleated and the other eye should be treated with radiation and chemotherapy.

Retinoblastoma may occur in more than one child in the same family and there is a high incidence of this tumor in the offspring of patients who have been successfully treated. These points should be considered in the overall management of the patient and his family.

WILMS' TUMOR

Wilms' tumor (nephroblastoma) is the only common malignant tumor of the kidney in the childhood age group. Although usually limited to one kidney, bilateral tumors have been reported in 5–10% of cases. Histologically, there may be marked variation from case to case. Abortive tubules and glomeruli are nearly always demonstrated.

Muscle fibers, adipose tissue, cartilage, bone, blood vessels, undifferentiated spindle cells and cuboidal epithelial cells are frequently noted.

Wilms' tumor usually has its clinical onset prior to five years of age but it may first become manifest during late childhood or adult life. The early course is characterized by the appearance of an asymptomatic mass in one side of the abdomen. During this stage, the tumor can often be felt by careful abdominal palpation at a time when the chances of successful treatment are good.

As the disease progresses, metastatic lesions usually appear in the lung parenchyma and there may be "seeding" of the tumor throughout the abdominal cavity. Hypertension is occasionally noted and hematuria occurs in a small percentage of cases. Metastatic lesions in bone and bone marrow are not frequent.

An intravenous pyelogram should be carried out as soon as possible after a mass has been noted in the area of the kidney. In the case of a Wilms' tumor, this will usually reveal some distortion of the renal pelvis or calyceal system. There may be little, if any, displacement of the kidney itself. This may be of value in ruling out a suprarenal mass, such as a neuroblastoma or adrenal cortical tumor.

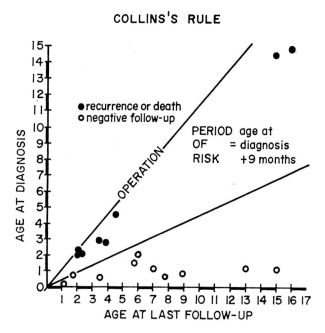

Chart 19. Indicates that at the time of diagnosis and treatment, the child has a period of risk for recurrence, should the child survive a similar period of time. (For instance, 9 months gestation plus his age at surgery, e.g., 9 months of age [should the child be able to survive 18 months without evidence of recurrence] then the child in all probability is a cure.)

A bone marrow examination may also be helpful in distinguishing a Wilms' tumor from a neuroblastoma. Extrinsic cells are rarely observed in cases of Wilms' tumor but are quite commonly seen in children with neuroblastoma.

The treatment of children with Wilms' tumor depends upon the extent of the disease at the time of the diagnosis. In those instances in which the tumor is well-localized and encapsulated, surgical excision should be done as soon as is practical. At the time of the surgical exploration, the opposite kidney should be examined in order that bilateral disease will not be missed. Postoperative radiation therapy to the tumor bed is administered in most clinics. However, decisions concerning radiation should be made on an individual basis.

If the tumor is localized, but unresectable, radiation therapy, chemotherapy or a combination of these two modalities should be administered in an effort to reduce the tumor to an extent that it can be completely excised.

In those instances in which there are distant metastases, palliation, and rarely a long-term survival, can be achieved at times by the use of radiation therapy, chemotherapy with actinomycin D or vincristine sulfate, or a combination of these two modalities. Occasionally, it is worthwhile to consider resection of a solitary pulmonary metastatic lesion but decision concerning this is usually made on an individual basis.

In children with bilateral Wilms' tumor, the goals of treatment are complete eradication of all neoplastic tissue and preservation of the maximal amount of normal kidney. Although these goals are rarely obtained there have been a few reported cases in which long survival resulted from surgical excision alone or surgical excision followed by radiation therapy.

The prognosis for long-term survival is good if there are no signs or symptoms of disease during the two years following treatment of a Wilms' tumor.

RHABDOMYOSARCOMA

In recent years rhabdomyosarcoma has become recognized as one of the more common malignant tumors of childhood. This is thought to be related to better diagnostic acumen and not to an increased incidence of the tumor. In the past it has often been misdiagnosed as a different type of malignant tumor, a benign tumor or an infectious process.

Histologically, the tumor in childhood is most often the embryonal type as contrasted to the pleomorphic, or adult, variety. A variety of cell types may be seen, including small round cells, spindle cells, elongated cells, cells with abundant eosinophilic cytoplasm and cells containing cross or longitudinal striations. If there is extension of the tumor into an orifice or cavity, it usually assumes a polypoid or myxomatous appearance.

Rhabdomyosarcoma may occur at any age throughout childhood. It begins most commonly in the soft tissues of the head or neck. Less common sites of origin are the urogenital area and long muscles of the back or extremities. A characteristic morphological type of rhabdomyosarcoma is the sarcoma botryoides which usually arises from the vagina, cervix or bladder and has a typical grapelike appearance grossly.

Clinically, the onset is usually characterized by the appearance of a nontender swelling which has a benign appearance. There is often considerable enlargement of the mass before the seriousness of the condition is appreciated. Extension of the tumor is either by direct invasion of contiguous tissue, by way of the blood stream to bone, bone marrow and lung parenchyma or by lymphatic channels. Metastases may occur early or the tumor may remain localized for many months.

The diagnosis of rhabdomyosarcoma can be strongly suspected from the clinical appearance and location of the tumor. Roentgenograms may reveal destructive lesions of adjacent bone or metastatic lesions in the lungs or distant bones. A bone marrow examination may reveal tumor cells (rhabdomyoblasts) which can be helpful not only for diagnosis but also for determining the extent of disease. Microscopic examination of biopsy material from the tumor will usually show enough findings to make a specific diagnosis. However, in those instances in which the histological appearance is not diagnostic, a recently developed immunofluorescence test for myosin (using fluorescin-labelled antimyosin antibodies) may help clarify the tissue.

The ideal treatment of a rhabdomyosarcoma is wide surgical excision. If the tumor has originated in one of the long muscles of the back or extremity, the entire muscle bundle should be removed.

Unfortunately, complete excision is rarely possible because of the location of the tumor. In those instances in which the tumor is localized, but unresectable, an attempt should be made to reduce the size with radiation therapy or chemotherapy (actinomycin D, vincristine sulfate, cyclophosphamide) or a combination of these modalities in order that surgical excision might be possible.

In children with distant metastases from a rhabdomyosarcoma, some palliation can be obtained by the use of chemotherapy with actinomycin D, vincristine sulfate or cyclophosphamide.

HODGKIN'S DISEASE

Hodgkin's disease occurs much less frequently in children than in adults. It is extremely rare under the age of 5 years, most cases having the onset in the preadolescent and adolescent years.

Clinically, the disease is characterized by the appearance of non-tender, firm, enlarged lymph nodes. These usually appear first in the neck but lymph nodes in any part of the body may be involved. As the disease progresses, multiple nodes appear and there is a tendency for these to be matted. Enlargement of the liver and spleen, fever, itching and skin rash are usually indications of advanced disease.

The diagnosis is made by examination of biopsy material from one of the involved lymph nodes. Early in the course the microscopic findings are frequently non-specific and can be consistent with "chronic infection" or "reactive hyperplasia." However, as the disease progresses varying degrees of pleomorphism, necrosis, fibrosis and eosinophilia appear. The pathognomonic finding is, of course, the Reed-Sternberg cell. This can usually be demonstrated in the moderately advanced cases but may not be seen early. Non-specific changes in the bone marrow (increased numbers of eosinophils, basophils and megakaryocytes) are a common finding.

The treatment and prognosis of Hodgkin's disease depends upon the clinical stage of the disease at the time of diagnosis.

Stage I disease indicates involvement of only one lymph node group. The treatment of choice in this situation is radiation therapy. It is important that an adequate tumor dose (3000–4000 r) be administered and that a radiation port with a wide margin be used. With this treatment the prognosis for long-term survival is good.

Stage II disease indicates involvement of lymph nodes in two or more contiguous areas of the body, all of the disease being either above or below the diaphragm. The treatment of choice in this situation is also radiation therapy as in Stage I disease. The prognosis is guarded but palliation can usually be obtained for a few years and there will be an occasional long-term survival.

Stage III disease indicates generalized involvement. Some palliation can be achieved by the use of chemotherapy with one of the vinca alkaloids, and by the use of radiation therapy for specific indications. However, the prognosis for long-term survival is poor and most patients with generalized disease have expired within three years from the time of the original diagnosis.

LYMPHOSARCOMA

Lymphosarcoma in childhood is classified according to the predominant cell type as either lymphocytic lymphosarcoma or reticulum cell sarcoma.

Lymphocytic lymphosarcoma is characterized clinically by the progressive enlargement of lymph nodes which are firm and not tender. These usually appear first in the cervical area but may have their origin in the axillary, inguinal, retroperitoneal, mesenteric or mediastinal nodes. There are usually no symptoms associated with these enlarged nodes unless they produce pressure on a structure such as the airway or the gastrointestinal tract. As the disease progresses, however, there is invasion of many tissues of the body.

Microscopic examination of the involved lymph node reveals obliteration of the normal architecture. There is diffuse infiltration of the gland with large dark-staining lymphocytes or by lymphoblasts of fairly uniform size. There is little or no tendency to pleomorphism.

The treatment of choice for most localized lymphocytic lymphosarcomas is radiation therapy. As in the case of Hodgkin's disease, an adequate tumor dose (3000–4000 r) and a radiation port with a wide margin should be used. With this treatment the prognosis is guarded but there are occasional long-term survivals. In rare instances, such as localized involvement in the abdomen, surgical excision may result in complete eradication of the malignancy.

Generalized lymphosarcoma is usually rapidly progressive and downhill. Some transient palliation can be obtained by the use of chemotherapy (steroids, alkylating agents, vinca alkaloids, antimetabolites), and by the use of radiation for specific indications. Terminally, however, conversion into acute lymphocytic leukemia is a common event.

Reticulum cell sarcoma is much less common in children than is lymphocytic lymphosarcoma. However, the clinical findings are essentially the same and the two diseases can only be differentiated by microscopic examination. In reticulum cell sarcoma the cells are larger and less uniform and varying amounts of reticulum can be demonstrated by the use of special stains.

The treatment and prognosis of reticulum cell sarcoma are the same as that for lymphocytic lymphosarcoma. However, terminal conversion into leukemia is not as common.

BONE TUMORS

Osteogenic sarcoma, although rare, is the most common malignant bone tumor of childhood. The clinical onset is most often in the adolescent or preadolescent age period. The most common site of origin is the metaphysis of one of the long bones, most commonly the femur or tibia. Rarely, this tumor arises from a flat bone such as the ilium.

The clinical course is characterized by slowly progressive swelling over the involved area and by slight or moderate pain and tenderness. Early in its course there are usually minimal signs and symptoms. As the disease progresses, however, there is usually a spread to the lungs and progressive signs of respiratory embarrassment.

The roentgenographic appearance is usually, but not always, highly suggestive of osteogenic sarcoma. There is evidence of bone destruction, periosteal new bone formation and a soft tissue mass. Occasionally a pathological fracture is present.

A biopsy of the lesion is necessary for a specific diagnosis. Microscopically there is evidence of tumor bone formation associated with pleomorphic stromal cells. A large amount of cartilage is frequently observed. Occasionally more than one biopsy is needed in order to be certain of the diagnosis.

The treatment of osteogenic sarcoma is surgical amputation through the bone proximal to the involved area. Radiation therapy and chemotherapy are usually of little value in the management of children with this tumor. Although there have been occasional cures of osteogenic sarcoma following early amputation, the survival rate is less than 10 percent in most large series of cases.

Ewing's sarcoma is the second most common malignant bone tumor of childhood. It occurs most commonly in the adolescent or preadolescent age group. However, it can also occur in younger children and is more common in children under 10 years of age than is osteogenic sarcoma. The most common sites of origin are the long bones, particularly the femur and tibia. However, it can arise from such flat bones as the ribs, scapula and those of the pelvis.

The early clinical findings of Ewing's sarcoma are those of swelling, slight pain and tenderness over the involved area. Fever may be present but this is usually associated with advanced disease. As the tumor progresses, metastases develop in the lungs, other bones and liver.

The roentgenographic appearance of Ewing's sarcoma is characterized by bone destruction, mottled radiolucencies and discontinuity of the cortex. There may be elevation of the periosteum with a resulting Codman's triangle. Periosteal new bone formation may give the so-called "onion-skin appearance." Moderate or marked soft-tissue swelling is frequently noted.

Microscopic examination reveals cells of uniform size which contain oval or round dark-staining nuclei and vacuolated cytoplasm. Pseudorosettes may be present and there may be considerable amounts of necrotic tissue and reactive bone formation. The overall histological appearance may be quite similar to that of infection, other primary tumors or metastatic disease, particularly neuroblastoma.

The treatment of choice of Ewing's sarcoma is radiation therapy to the entire length of the involved bone. In these cases in which metastases has occurred, transient palliation can be obtained by the use of chemotherapy (alkylating agents, vinca alkaloids) and by radiation therapy. However, the prognosis is extremely poor and the survival rate is less than 5% in most reported series.

Suggested Reading

James, David H., Jr.: Summary for St. Jude's Tumor Therapy Hospital, Memphis, Tenn.

Owings, Richard S., and Radakovich, Michael: Wilms' Tumor: An Evaluation of Prognosis and Treatment, *Surgery, 46*:5, 1959.

Owings, Richard S.: Recent Advances in Pediatric Surgery, *J Med A Ga, 52*:3, March, 1963.

MISCELLANEOUS TUMORS

Lipoblastoma

Six patients with lipoblastoma have been reported since Van Meurs first described his case of "embryonic lipoma" (Van Meurs, 1947). Because this tumor has not been reported in American clinical literature, and since lipoblastomas, because of their locally infiltrative nature, might be confused with a malignancy, we felt that a review of the literature and report of the two cases which have occurred during recent years at the Children's Hospital of Philadelphia would be timely.

Lipoblastoma is a lipoid neoplasm of infancy which is composed of numerous lipoblasts arranged in a loose, myxomatous stroma with irregular fetal fat lobules and without bizarre appearing cells. Despite its active lipogenesis and tendency to recur locally, it does not metastasize.

Van Meurs reported a five-month old patient with transformation of an embryonic lipoma of the thigh to a common lipoma. Three months after initial surgery local recurrence necessitated re-operation. During the twenty month post-operative period following the initial excision, local recurrences prompted four such surgical attempts at extirpation. The final biopsy, twenty months post-operatively, had the histologic appearance of mature adipose tissue.

Bellious described an eight-month old girl with a history of enlargement of the right arm and forearm over a five-week period (Bellious, F., Beaz, J., Shumacker, H. E., 1958). The right upper extremity was larger than the left but was not increased in length. There was pink discoloration of the entire extremity. A soft swelling occupied the right pectoral region and axilla. There was no associated limitation of motion or pain. At operation, the tumor diffusely involved the subcutaneous tissue and deep structures of the thorax, neck and axilla. The mass partially encompassed the axillary artery and vein as well as the brachial plexus. This was dissected free without injury to these structures but gross tumor remained. Despite incomplete removal, tumor growth has not been evident in the ensuing three years.

Kauffman, reporting on 27 lipoid tumors in children, had four patients with lipoblastoma (Kauffman, S.L., Stout, A.P., 1959). These all occurred in infants less than one year of age. In each case, the duration of awareness of a tumor was short; one infant had a mass that had grown to 8 cm in diameter after being barely noticeable two weeks prior to its removal. The parents of this four and one-half month old girl described a lump overlying the clavicle which appeared "overnight." At operation, two weeks following its appearance, the tumor measured 3 cm in diameter. Three months later it reappeared and was excised. The child has been clinically free of tumor for a four month follow-up period. The location of tumors in these four patients were: the neck and mediastinum; the arm and axilla; the buttocks; and the chest wall. In the latter case, three months following initial surgery a local recurrence was noted in the chest wall. The duration of follow-up in these four patients was from four months to two and one-half years with tumor recurring locally in only one case. Stout states that lipoblastoma is a benign tumor and recurs only when incompletely excised.

L.F. was admitted to the Children's Hospital of Philadelphia at 16 months of age with a soft, circumscribed 4x4x4 cm mass in the right popliteal region. At surgery, the tumor had a fatty, lobulated appearance with a pseudocapsule; it was excised and transected at the point where the tumor disappeared into the joint capsule. After a twenty-six month follow-up, there is no evidence of recurrence.

E.P. is an 18-month-old infant admitted with a two-month history of gradual enlargement of the right thigh and calf. Two weeks prior to admission a firm mass had been noted in the right groin which on exploration measured 5x7x7 cm and had a firm, fatty, lobulated appearance. The tumor jammed into the femoral canal and the obturator foramen, and with some difficulty was dissected free of its femoral canal attachments. At its deepest point it was necessary to transect the tumor where it departed into the obturator canal. Six weeks following surgery a large mass was again evident in the right femoral area. The mass was again resected and eighteen months following this procedure the infant was clinically free of tumor.

These tumors both had the appearance of well differentiated lipoblastomas.

In evaluating the literature together with our own patients with lipoblastoma, certain clinical points are worth noting. All patients with lipoblastoma were sixteen months of age or under and no deaths occurred. The appearance of the tumor in three patients was of only two weeks' duration. The duration of the tumor as well as recurrences have been short suggesting a fast tumor growth rate. Limb enlargement has not previously been highlighted but antedated the appearance of the tumor in two patients, one of ours and one in the literature. A lipoid tumor was evident by x-ray in both cases here reported suggesting that

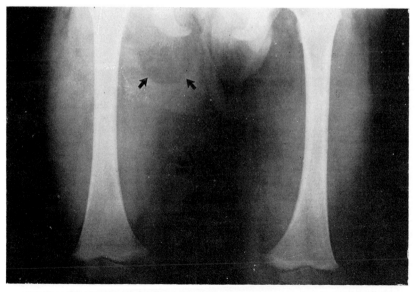

Figure 1. The radiolucency seen in the soft tissue film suggest a lipoid tumor in patients with lipoblastoma.

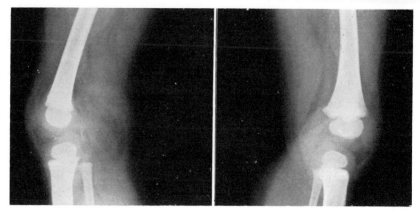

Figure 2.   The radiolucency seen in the soft tissue film suggest a lipoid tumor in patients with lipoblastoma.

this is a very useful diagnostic adjunct. Despite Stout's statement that incomplete excision is followed by local recurrence, of four patients in which total excision was not accomplished, recurrences occurred in only two patients. It is hoped that increased awareness of benign nature of this malignant-appearing tumor will prevent unnecessary radical procedures such as amputation.

Suggested Reading

Bellious, F. Beaz, J. Schumacker, H. E.: *Am J Path, 34*:1149, 1958.
Kauffman, S. L., and Stout, A. P.: *Cancer, 12*:912, 1959.
Van Meurs, V. P.: *Brit J Surg, 34*:282, 1947.
Owings, Koop, *et al.:* International College of Surgeons, 1966.

LYMPHOHEMANGIOMA

This tumor is associated with thrombocytopenia and often has other hematological problems such as AHG deficiency. The patient may present as a pseudohemophiliac. A splenectomy does not relieve the thrombocytopenia. The afferent vessels to the tumor have a higher platelet count than the efferent vessels and evidently the platelets are sequestrated in the tumor. With total removal of the tumor, the platelet count immediately returns to normal and, at the same time, the AHG deficiency is corrected.

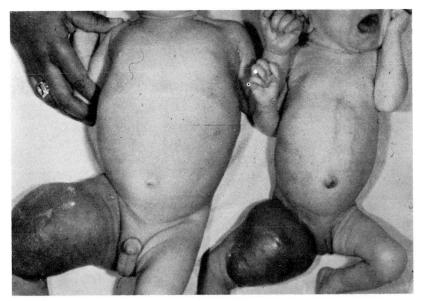

Figure 3. These giant reddish rapidly-growing tumors trap platelets.

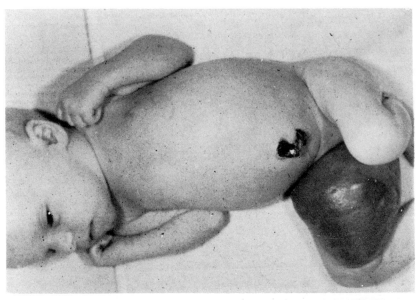

Figure 4. These giant tumors often have an associated AHG deficiency.

Chapter 15

TRACHEO-ESOPHAGEAL FISTULAS

One is not infrequently confronted with the question of who should operate on patients with tracheo-esophageal fistulas. I would answer that question by saying that the person who should operate is any person who is prepared to deal with all possible ramifications that may be associated with not only the technical aspects of the several approaches to the tracheo-esophageal fistulas (depending on the problem) but also the associated defects which may lead to immediate post-operative difficulties. I have had the experience of seeing an anesthesiologist unfamiliar with the problem set up a "closed system" without the stomach first being vented with a gastrostomy. Since the most common type of T.E. fistula is associated with a lower esophageal connection with the bronchus, this could lead to over-distention of the stomach and perforation. In approximately 10% of the patients with T.E. fistula, there is an associated imperforate anus; approximately 10% of the patients develop pyloric stenosis post-operatively; whether this is due to vagal injury or some vagal defect associated with the primary defect is unknown. This author has operated on 13 T.E. fistulas with 9 survivors.

One technique that has been highlighted by Dr. Luther Longino is that of a retropleural approach through the back. This technique is particularly useful in the small premature and avoids an open thoracotomy.

The pre-operative use of a trans-nasal, upper esophageal sump suction is valuable in preventing excessive pulmonary aspiration. This is achieved by threading a small polyethelene tube into the side of a larger naso-gastric tube to allow for the presence of air in the upper obstructed esophageal pouch.

One report from a well-known clinic reports that of 12 T.E.

fistulas operated there were 11 deaths. Ten different surgeons performed the procedures. The only surviving patient was operated by the surgeon who had previously performed one case. This would certainly indicate that the surgeon with the most experience with the problem and who is prepared to stay with the child constantly during the post-operative period is certainly the one of choice to perform the surgery.

Suggested Reading

Clatworthy, H. W., Jr.: Esophageal Atresia, Importance of Early Diagnosis and Treatment, *Pediatrics, 16*:122, 1955.

Chapter 16

LYE INGESTION

Probably the greatest injustice to the care of the child who ingests lye is the use of hydrocortisone in the acute care period. The esophagus is lined by stratified squamous epithelium and, in cases of first or second degree burn of the esophagus or of the skin, it makes little difference what application is used in that the stratified squamous epithelium heals with little or no scarring. On the other hand, in cases of third degree burn of the esophagus or the skin, cortisone will have no effect on the amount of scarring.

Since the esophagus is at its strongest immediately following the injury, it is the author's policy to perform an immediate esophagoscopy to obtain a visual evaluation of the extent of damage. Marked swelling usually indicates third degree damage. If complete obstruction of the esophagus appears imminent, a small silicone naso-gastric tube is introduced into the stomach for future feedings. The child is placed on antibiotics prophylactically since there is often aspiration with chemical pneumonitis. Dilitations are instituted at four day intervals with the intervals progressively increased as the child's esophagus dilates. If long segments of the esophagus have third degree burns making dilitations hazardous, it may be necessary to perform a gastrostomy and attempt dilitation in retrograde fashion. If this is impossible, the colon may be sterilized and an interposition colon transplant performed similar to the procedure described by Dr. C. Everett Koop for bleeding varices. If a colon interposition is necessary, it is highly important to perform a Hinecke-Mickulicz pyloroplasty also since the vagus nerves are usually injured with resulting associated pylorospasm.

Suggested Reading

Gellis, S. S., and Holt, L. E., Jr.: The Treatment of Lye Ingestion, Salzer Method, *Ann Otol Rhinol Larynogol, 51*:1086, 1942.

Holinger, P. H., *et al.:* The Conservative and Surgical Management of Benign Strictures of the Esophagus, *J Thoracic Surg, 28*:345, 1954.

Chapter 17

SIMILARITY BETWEEN PATIENT WITH DIAPHRAGMATIC HERNIA AND OMPHALOCELE

In both diaphragmatic hernia and omphalocele, the peritoneal cavity does not contain the full volume of the viscera and the attempt to place the entire viscera into this underdeveloped cavity may be disastrous. Dr. Meeker highlighted the very important point that in cases of diaphragmatic hernia one may actually have to create an omphalocele and place the bowel in a skin enclosure; to decrease the pressure on the inferior vena cava and to avoid "splinting" the diaphragm. Dr. Edward Free has shown that in cases in which the inferior vena cava pressure is in the range of 12 mm of water or above, the outlook is very poor; therefore, in both these conditions it is very important to monitor the inferior vena cava pressure during surgical repair with an indwelling catheter. In both of these conditions, the bowel is not rotated into the abdomen. Usually, there is an associated malrotation of the bowel with the possibility of ensuing complications associated with this condition.

In summary, in both diaphragmatic hernia and omphalocele the bowel is not rotated into the abdomen—therefore, there is the condition of malrotation and the possibility of volvulus. Often, the peritoneal cavity is not large enough to accommodate the viscera—this should be of prime concern to the surgeon. The simple closure of the skin may be the most desirable procedure for both conditions, after reduction and closure of the diaphragmatic defect. An indwelling catheter should be placed in the inferior vena cava through the saphenous bulb to monitor the pressure following the surgical closure of each defect. On occasion, this author has performed a left lobectomy of the liver to increase the space available in the peritoneal cavity. The left lobe of the liver of the newborn is roughly ⅓ of the liver volume whereas in the adult it is roughly ¼ of the liver volume—therefore, a large amount of space may be gained by a left lobectomy. A left lobectomy is a relatively simple procedure requiring placement of mattress sutures to the right of the falciforme ligament for hemostasis. An additional procedure which has been widely publicized is the use of a teflon sac, either inside the skin or attached to the skin, for a limited period of time—and gradually decreasing the size of the sac as the abdomen acclimates to more of the viscera. The treatment of both these conditions is one of continuing advancement in percentage of success. The mortality and morbidity has steadily decreased with the increasing awareness of the major problems. To quote one prominent surgeon, "one cannot put two pounds of worms in a one pound sac." If one makes every effort to avoid splinting the diaphragm, obstructing the inferior vena cava, and to allow the abdominal cavity to acclimate gradually to the size of the viscera (mindful that post-op volvulus due to malrotation is a distinct possibility), the percentage of survival should continue to increase.

Suggested Reading

Avery, M. E.: *The Lung and Its Disorders in the Newborn Infant,* W. B. Saunders Co., Philadelphia, 1964.

Chapter 18

DIAPHRAGMATIC HERNIA

The patient with a diaphragmatic hernia has several associated problems: First of all, the bowel is not rotated properly. Therefore, there is associated malrotation with the possibility of a volvulus. The second factor is that usually the left pleural space is the site of the hernia and the lung has not been able to develop and is hypoplastic. This particular condition will generally correct itself within 2–3 weeks following surgical correction of the hernia. Under no circumstances should the anesthesiologist put over 15 mm of water pressure to try to expand the lung. If the infant is cyanotic, not only should a well-working nasogastric tube be introduced for G.I. decompression, but correction of the acidosis with bicarbonate is urgently desirable to decrease the acidemia associated with anaerobic respiration. Following acid base correction, the defect should be corrected and the bowel re-introduced into the abdomen, being careful not to increase the inferior vena cava pressure beyond 12 cm of water. This indicates that one should have a transsaphenous bulb vena-cava catheter in place to check this pressure. Should the liver be in the chest, the prognosis is poorer but one may want to do a wedge resection of the left lobe of the liver to give more space. This is highly desirable in large defects to effect the closure of the abdomen which just involves the skin so as not to put increased pressure on the inferior vena cava, and also to avoid splinting the diaphragm.

The importance of correcting the metabolic acidosis pre-operatively, as well as creating a ventral hernia sufficient to allow for a 12 cm or less vena cava pressure cannot be over emphasized.

Suggested Reading

Denes, J., *et al.: J Ped Surg*, 2:359–63, Aug. 1967.

Eraklis, *et al.: J Ped Surg,* 2:354–358.
Vaughn, C. C.: *Dis Chest, 54*:467, Nov. 1968.
Rastich, M. M., *et al.: Arch Surg, 64*:794.
Wolfson, S. A., *et al.: Surgery, 24*:846.
Murphy, D. R., *et al.: Am J Surg, 101*:581–587.

Chapter 19

OMPHALOCELE

Facts determining the prognosis in an infant with an omphalocele are:

(1) The size of the sac.
(2) The presence or absence of liver in the sac.
(3) Whether there has been a rupture of the sac or,
(4) Co-existing malrotations.
(5) Whether the bowel has been kept decompressed.
(6) Whether there is associated prematurity.
(7) Whether an early operation is undertaken.

Small or low omphaloceles may be associated with extrophy of the urogenital plate. In 45 infants reported by Jones, P.G. (*Arch Dis Child, 38*:180–187, 1963) serious malformations were present in 35 and were the direct or indirect cause of death in 21 infants. Fourteen had less serious malformations. Malrotation of the bowel is frequently an accompanying defect. If one merely closes the skin over the defect and leaves an inferior-vena-cava pressure of less than 12 cm of water, the chance are in favor of survival. In some instances, the method of Drs. Gross and Shuster using a teflon bag with skin closure is desirable followed by cinching up of the bag to decrease the defect at approximately 10-day intervals as the abdomen acclimates to the bowel. In three instances, the author has removed the left lobe of the liver as an adjunct to closing the defect and this has given the necessary space to be able to close the skin primarily without undue tension.

Suggested Reading

Jones, P. G.: *Arch Dis Child., 38*:180–187; 1963.

Kieswetter, W. B.: Neonatal Surgical Conditions Incompatible with
   Life without Surgical Correction. *Pennsylvania M.J., 59*:791, 1956
Gross, R. E.: *The Surgery of Infancy and Childhood.* Philadelphia,
   W. B. Saunders Co., 1953.

Chapter 20

MUCOVISCIDOSIS

Chronologically speaking, mucovisidosis and its complications follow a rather predictable pattern. Prior to birth, the presence of *polyhydramnios* is often indicative of meconium ileus. *Meconium ileus* is one of the most common causes of intestinal obstruction. The polyhydramnios is thought to be due to the presence of meconium which obstructs the swallowed amniotic fluid from reaching the terminal ilium and colon for reabsorption into the fetal, and maternal, circulation. Thus, the accumulation of amniotic fluid.

The presence of *calcium in the x-ray of the peritoneal cavity* should made one suspect mucovisidosis with associated meconium ileus and *perforation*. Approximately 70% of the patients with meconium ileus have *volvulus* to some degree. The presence of *meconium plug syndrome* or the early occurrence of *rectal prolapse* is frequently indicative of mucovisidosis.

Following relief of the meconium ileus, attention should be centered on *nutrition*. The use of Cotazyme, a balanced mixture of proteolytic enzymes and lipases, is very helpful in improving nutrition and absorption of fats and proteins. There are various degrees of mucovisidosis and from the author's experience the children who develop wheezing in the first six months have the more severe disease whereas those who have *respiratory problems* after six months have a better prognosis. Following the nutritional problem, the respiratory problems occur. There is often *sweating before age three months* which is highly suspect of this condition. The respiratory difficulties are major and result in recurrent Staph infections (and Pseudomonas) which may require extra efforts in bronchial toilet and insulfation of antibiotics locally, as well as, rotation of antibiotics p.o. Following the protein wasting, *cirrhosis* frequently develops as does pancreatic scar-

104

ring. With cirrhosis for prolonged periods—around the sixth year there may be upper *G.I. bleeding associated with esophageal varices.* With survival of these patients into the teens, the pancreas may have enough islet cell damage to result in *diabetes.* Patients, especially in the teens, often demonstrate *mental changes*—probably associated with chronic illness and resentment. They often have the immature and obstreperous personalities similar to that seen in the teenage diabetic.

The trans-nasogastric biopsy of the intestinal mucosa, described by Dr. Schwachman, has been a real advance. Other members of the family may have the mucosal, microscopic changes typical of mucovisidosis even though they do not have the overt disease.

In cystic fibrosis, there is an increased quantity of sodium, potassium and chloride lost in sweat. Factors that may increase the sweat levels in addition to a heat load are adrenal insufficiency, ectodermal dysplasia, malnutrition, allergic disease, bronchiectasis, and diabetes. Genetic factors may also play a part in that certain families have a tendency toward excessive sweating. An increase in salt and nitrogen intake may increase sweat levels as well as the poor general physical condition with exercise or unusual climatic conditions.

The sodium and chloride content of sweat increases progressively with age. Potassium concentration does not vary with age.

The iontophoresis sweat electrolyte determination is valid from birth, chloride contents of 60 mEq per liter, or more, is most suggestive of the diagnosis.

Suggested Reading

Anderson, C. M., and Freeman, M.: "Sweat Test" Results in Normal Persons of Different Ages Compared with Families with Fibrocystic Disease of the Pancreas. *Arch Dis Child, 35*:518, 1960.

Shwachman, H., and Leubner, H.: Mucovisidosis, *Advances in Pediatrics, 7*:249, 1955.

Barnett, H. L.: *Pediatrics,* 15th Ed., Appleton, Century, Croft, 1972.

Nelson, W. E., Vaughan, V. C., and McKay, R. J.: *Textbook of Pediatrics,* 9th Ed., W. B. Saunders Co., 1969, p. 855–867.

Chapter 21

MECONIUM ILEUS

Meconium Ileus is one of the two conditions in which the new-born is *distended at the time of birth*. In fetal distress, there may be acute gastric distention associated with ingestion of amniotic fluid and blood. An x-ray of the abdomen immediately shows differentiation between these two conditions. In meconium ileus, there are irregular sized loops of bowel that show fluid levels. In simple gastric distention, the bowel caliber is normal and uniform.

In some series, 70% of the infants with meconium ileus had an associated volvulus. Therefore, laparotomy after proper preparation and hydration of the patient is essential. Most of these infants have a water, sodium and chloride deficit—probably associated with intra-uterine emesis. Of the various procedures that have been described (enterotomy with irrigation with hydrogen peroxide or 2% Hyaluronidase; loop or catheter enterostomy; resection of the distended bowel with end-to-end or side-to-side anastomosis; Mickulicz ileo-colostomy or Mickulicz double ileostomy; loop enterostomy of the distended bowel), the author believes the procedure of choice to produce the least shock and lowest mortality in the majority of cases is the use of the loop ileostomy of the distended bowel. This allows for inspection of the bowel and relief of the volvulus which usually is associated. It avoids peritoneal contamination and is the least shocking procedure. It also allows for staging of further procedures such as irrigation of the loop for relief of meconium obstruction. This method provides a sure method of relieving the obstruction immediately; prevents trauma and possible shock; avoids peritoneal contamination and allows for post-operative irrigation of the inspissated meconium. One must be aware of the considerable amounts of fluid and electrolyte loss that will require replacement associated with the early bowel activity with an enterostomy.

Within 7–10 days the bowel is usually completely open and one can then restore the continuity of the bowel.

Suggested Reading

White, Harvey: Meconium Ileus—New Roentgen Sign. *Radiology,* 66:567, 1956.

Chapter 22

PEPTIC ULCER

Peptic ulcers in children are being seen much more frequently and suspected by the pediatrician and the general practitioner. Duodenal ulcers outnumber gastric ulcers six to one and in one series ten to one (*The Pediatric Patient*, 1964).

In children, the pattern is much less specific than that seen in the adult in that the pain does not have the two to three hour postprandial characteristics. The pain is vague and more generalized in children and may be caused by any food—even foods that ordinarily might be expected to relieve the pain. With modern x-ray techniques, the diagnosis should be highly suspect. Many children have a fast transit time through the duodenum and with increased pylorospasm one may have to be satisfied (although some may disagree) with the ulcer being strongly suspect rather than necessarily demonstrating a crater. In x-ray studies of children's stomachs who complain of vague abdominal pain, an ulcer incidence of 10% has been found. The disease is more prevalent in boys than in girls. In one series by Berg *et al.* (*The Pediatric Patient*, 1964), in a population of 100,000 people, 255 cases of ulcer in children were found in a one-year period. Of these, 145 boys and 110 were girls. Duodenal ulcers numbered 229 to the number of gastric ulcers which was 26.

An ulcer tendency exists among children of the same family. In Berg's series, in a case of a 5-year-old, there were 3 siblings, the parents, and an uncle, with peptic ulcers. In this series, a family history of ulcer was found in 24% of the 255 reported cases. Prouty found that the majority of patients had at least one parent with an ulcer. In the newborn, the incidence of ulcer was much more common in the premature and perforation occurred in a high proportion. Two-thirds of the diagnosed cases showed signs of internal bleeding. Some rejected feedings and failed to thrive. The symptoms are highly variable in the infant and young child. The most common complaints are vague abdominal pain, mild tenderness, frequent nausea, anorexia, and acid eructation together with occasional early morning vomiting. Conspicuously, as noted earlier, pain is frequently aggravated by meals and rarely relieved by eating. Many children give a history of feeding often. One must frequently distinguish between other abdominal conditions which may be associated with vague abdominal pain such as pyelonephritis and other causes of duodenitis such as nasal respiratory allergy with copious post-nasal swallowing of mucous. In making the diagnosis, it is important that the radiologist be patient and take at least eight to twelve spot films. We might mention in passing that it often is the impression that an individual with a nasal respiratory allergy seems to have a much higher incidence of peptic ulcer. Other stressful conditions are well known to be causative of peptic ulcer such as CNS lesions, malnutrition, failure to thrive, burns and any debilitating chronic disease. Gastric outlet obstructions such as pyloric stenosis have been reported to have a subsequent higher family history of ulcer. The long-term use of steroids greatly favors the development of peptic ulcer. The fearful, "high-strung" child who lives in a so-called high-tension family and is apt to have behavior problems and to suffer from anxiety is much more prone to this illness.

Some of the associated findings are a history of fear of school, morning emesis, prolonged enuresis. In the case of the unusually stressful situation as well as in the instance of prolonged use of steroids, multiple ulcers are not uncommon. A medical regimen is indicated and generally will cure most ulcers. However, if the child has recurrent severe episodes of bleeding and/or signs of recurring partial gastric obstruction and has had a reasonable thorough medical management which has failed to keep the ulcer cured, then one should have no hesitation about undertaking surgery. Here again, the procedure of choice is a much simpler one in that usually a bilateral vagotomy and drainage procedure are all that is necessary. The drainage procedure of choice is pyloroplasty. If, as very rarely occurs, this is unsuccessful in keeping the ulcer cured, then one should have no hesitation about undertaking surgery. One may consider the possibility of an antrectomy.

It is important to remember that with recurrent severe ulcer symptoms the possibility of Ellison-Zollinger Syndrome may exist with an associated pancreatic carcinoma. This author has personally seen two patients (5 years and 8 years) with this syndrome.

Suggested Reading

Raffensperger, John G., *et al.: SG&O, 123*:1269, Dec. 1966.

Fisher, John H.: *Am J Dis Child, 50*:58, Jan. 1950.

Zollinger, R. M.: CPC with Discussion. *New Eng J Med, 262*:1132, Jan. 2, 1960.

Chapter 23

MISCELLANEOUS SUBJECTS

RESPIRATORY DISTRESS SYNDROME

Respiratory distress syndrome often accompanies congenital anomalies and prematurity.

J. P. Owen Thomas *et al.* have demonstrated that when respiratory distress syndrome exists and intermittent positive pressure is indicated, that failure to raise the arterial oxygen above 50 mm merc./Hg is generally associated with a grave prognosis. A prolonged expiration phase is desirable.

Pneumothorax must be anticipated as the most common surgical complication.

PEDIATRIC SURGICAL MAXIMS

The following maxims are from some of the leaders in pediatric surgery and reflect attitudes that have led to a great saving of life in the pediatric surgical patient:

Sir Lancelot Barrington Ward: *"Adults may be safely treated as children, but the converse can lead to disaster."* One can improvise for the adult much more safely than for the child. Illustrations of this: one would not hang up a 1000 cc bottle of I.V. fluid for an infant whose blood volume is 300 cc. This would be comparable to hanging up a 55 gallon drum of fluid for an adult. Until the past 15–20 years, the anesthesiologists in smaller hospitals have improvised with anesthesia equipment much to the detriment of the pediatric patient. The excessive dead space in some of the extensions of equipment for endotracheal anesthesia in adults can lead to disaster if used for an infant.

Dr. Robert Gross: *"Keep the infant dry."* Dr. Gross has emphasized the importance of staying on the minimum side of hydration. As emphasized elsewhere in this book the infant, in a high humidity atmosphere, needs very little fluid and can tolerate starvation quite well. Indeed, his weight tends to remain quite stable for the first several days following surgery. If one calculates fluid needs on the basis of the pediatric medical patient whose loss is usually copious due to vomiting and diarrhea the pediatric surgical patient will be grossly over-hydrated.

Dr. C. Everett Koop: *"Intelligent neglect"* in the handling of prematures. Nurses who are unfamiliar with the problems of the premature have difficulty in keeping their hands off of the seriously ill surgical infant. They will be in and out of the incubator every ten or fifteen minutes which is totally exhausting to the infant. The care of these patients must be organized so that the infant is disturbed only every 3–4 hours.

I believe it was Dr. Leonard Bockman, Chief of Pediatric Anesthesia at The Children's Hospital of Philadelphia, who pointed out to me that *over-distended bowel is slow to return.* Especially in upper intestinal problems with over-distended bowel there is a 4–6 day lag after relief of the obstruction before bowel function begins to return to normal. Any attempt to feed orally in these cases—especially if the naso-gastric drainage is still green or yellow —is useless.

Some of the maxims that I have used in teaching and have evolved from personal experience are the following:

"No Trendelenberg for long periods in the newborn." The newborn breathes largely through diaphragmatic action and the weight of the abdominal viscera in the Trendelenberg position is a tremendous burden. In this position, the infant may become exhausted and stop breathing.

"Monitor without handling." If one can monitor the infant's pulse and respiration without entering the incubator and physically disturbing the infant it is much superior in that it allows the infant to rest.

"Stage procedures." The surgeon may wish to accomplish the entire operative procedure at one sitting but one should ask "what is the immediate problem" and the surgery should be directed only at that specific need—especially since these patients are often already in a precarious condition. It is much better to do a little at a time with a live patient than accomplish the entire procedure and have the infant die within the post-operative period. An ex-

tension of this is *"do as little as necessary to control the problem."* An illustration of this is a patient who had duplication of most of the small bowel. The prime problem, however, was that the child's hemoglobin was 4 gm and was exsanguinating into this bowel. The bleeding point was identified but following this a great deal of time was lost in dissecting out the bowel to determine all aspects of the anatomy. The proper course of action would have been to control the bleeding and leave the other aspects to a later procedure when the child was in a better condition.

"Reaction to shock is already at the maximum during major surgery." The infant's pulse is in the range of perhaps 150–180 and he is able to increase his exchange volume very effectively only by increasing the rate. This is why a patient's chart may show that during anesthesia the signs remained the same and without sudden changes—due to the fact that the infant's response is already at the maximum levels.

"Blood replacement should be kept on a minute-to-minute basis, calculated on the weight of the sponges"—each soaked sponge containing approximately 10 cc of blood. The first indication of shock may be associated with poor capillary return to the ear or compression of the skin and subcutaneous tissue. A sudden overload of blood to circumvent shock may lead to pulmonary edema and, of course, it is far preferable to prevent shock than to have to treat it.

"Rule of 13" and *"Rule of 7"* for burns in babies. The "Rule of 13" is used for surface area estimates in infants instead of the usual 9–9–18 ratio for surface areas of adults—for instance instead of the head and neck being 9 as in the adult—in the infant it is 13% of the body surface; the two upper extremities are 13% of the infant's total surface and each lower extremity is 13%. This provides for an easy formula for estimating burns in babies. The "Rule of 7" is a method of anticipating the possible complications following an acute burn in an infant:

(1) Seven hours after the burn, if there has been inhalation of the flames, the infant will probably die due to pulmonary edema.

(2) Within 72 hours, if not vigorously supported, the infant is apt to die from irreversible shock.

(3) In 7 days, if not prevented, the infant may have severe difficulty from hyperkalemia and renal shutdown.

(4) At 7 weeks, the infant may encounter difficulties associated with overwhelming gram negative infection and failure to heal.

"Keep care simple." One is often appalled by the maze of orders that may be left for an acutely ill surgical infant. A simple routine which provides for intake and output and monitoring is all that can be performed safely without totally exhausting the infant.

"Simple pediatric chart procedures." A chart or any record should tell a story. One frequently sees reams and reams of wasted paper—in a hospital chart it may be totally impossible to find the important information in such a chart. A good chart needs vital signs, intake and output, and weight recorded all together in one simple form to allow the busy house officer to evaluate the progress of the patient at a glance. A dangerous practice is a nurse taking vital signs and recording them on a piece of paper slipped into her pocket until the end of her shift at which time she suddenly realizes the progressive degeneration of the patient which had been occurring. Signs must be recorded on the chart immediately after taking them in order to evaluate the direction of change and to recognize immediately any deterioration.

"The surgical loss of children and why." The usual reason for loss of a patient is due to failure to attend to the minute details. The operative procedure may be performed perfectly. However, if the patient has not been protected from hypothermia and acidemia and shock, the surgery accomplishes nothing.

"Pyloric position post-operatively." For some reason, the infant who is placed in a right decubitus position with head and chest elevated seems to empty his stomach better. Any gas bubble erupted will be up against the esophagus. Post-op abdominal surgical patients always seem to do better placed in this position. This is especially true after feedings are instituted and lessens the hazard of aspiration.

INTRA-UTERINE SURGERY

The interest and increased investigation in intra-uterine surgery and the high incidence of low birth weight in association with congenital anomalies make the subject of under-nutrition in the mother and fetus of interest to pediatric surgery. The rate of growth of the fetus is directly related to the size of the fetus at term and to the length of gestation as well as to the food supply—

primarily dependent upon the quality of maternal blood diffusing the placenta. Maternal under-nutrition probably does not reduce the size of the offspring. One cannot extrapolate the effects of under-nutrition on animals during gestation to that of humans. It is, however, of interest that the low birth weight infants are more common and infant mortality higher among mothers age 15–19 than in those over 25. Similarly, prematurity and high mortality rates are notoriously seen in unwed mothers and others who receive poor prenatal care. In measurements of growth, chemical factors as well as physical factors must be considered. The ratio of protein to DNA content of growing organs is under major investigation. Increase in cell division or hyperplasia is reflected by a proportionately greater increase in DNA within the cell whereas in hypertrophy of the cell there is proportionately greater increase in protein with little or no increase in DNA. Studies to date indicate that under-nutrition during hyperplasia will decrease the rate of cell division and lead to a permanent deficit in the number of cells in an organ. Under-nutrition during a phase of hypertrophy decreases the cell size only and is of a temporary nature. In this regard, under-nourished mice have been found to have both a decreased number of cells and decreased cytoplasm within the cell. The number of cerebral neurons in rats at birth is the final number. Offspring of low-protein fed rats had smaller bodies and smaller brains than the offspring of control groups. They also had a 10% fewer cerebral neurons and 10% less brain protein cells. Second generation rats of these low-protein fed rats, when kept on a normal diet throughout pregnancies, showed body and brain weights which were normal but the brain DNA and brain cell number were 13% lower than the second generation of controls. The effects of relatively mild chronic hypoxia on rats and mice are clearly more devastating than under-nutrition. This is probably also true in the human. A major problem is how to diagnose the presence of intra-uterine growth retardation. Rats exposed to cigarette smoke had a far greater fetal weight reduction than that associated with decrease in maternal food intake. It therefore, appears that cigarette tobacco smoke contains factors that retard fetal growth.

Metabolic rate growth per unit of body surface area is probably not a valid physiological constant but is probably more nearly related to energy production and metabolic rate in the individual cell population of the organ. The brain, liver, kidney and heart which account for only 6% of the total adult body weight contribute ⅔ of the total metabolic rate.

To ferret out the answers to the questions that arise, one must remember the admonition of Alexander Pope "the proper study of mankind is man." However, some of these animal studies no doubt apply in part to human growth. Rates of growth in both height and weight of animals and human infants were higher in warm raised subjects than in cool raised subjects. There are many unexplained factors such as why one infant is able to obtain more gain from a given amount of food than another which may be due to the great variation observed in oxygen consumption among newborn infants. It is known that amino acid crosses the blood-brain barrier more readily in the more immature animal. Of the variables, including environmental temperature, thyroid hormone, estrogens, respiratory acidosis—none have a striking effect on brain-protein synthesis except the environmental temperature. Isolated bits of information suggest that mobilization and oxidation of fatty acids before birth may constitute a significant energy source for the fetus. Rises in serum fatty acids in the viscera observed in human newborn are related to cold exposure rather than starvation. When severely obese adults lose weight, they do so by decreasing the amount of lipid per cell—not by reducing the total number of fat cells in the body. In obese children, however, there are not only larger fat cells but also a greater number of fat cells than in the non-obese child. The placenta, as an organ, plays an intimate part by its transfer differentiation. Essential fatty acids in fetal blood can be accounted for only on the basis of placental transfer. In deprivation studies of sodium or potassium in pregnant rats, the placenta is far more effective in protecting the fetus against maternal hypocalcemia than against maternal hyponatremia and hypokalemia. The healthy growing infant tends to be in a negative net acid balance. The less mature the infant the less fat is absorbed. The intestinal absorption of calcium decreases progressively in percentage as the intake of calcium is increased.

COMMENTS ON CYANOTIC CONGENITAL HEART DISEASE IN INFANCY

Cyanosis in infancy generally connotes, in order of frequency:

(1) A large ventricular septal defect, with equal pressures in the ventricules and this means a 1 cm square defect per square meter of body surface.

(2) Tetralogy of Fallot with a similar size defect. In this case, the child is born with normal color generally and develops cyanosis of an advancing nature over a 3–4 month period.

(3) Transposition of the great vessels.

Once the patient gets to the point where he is having cyanotic spells he is probably far advanced in his disease. In tetralogy, the most common pulmonary artery defect is a valvular defect with a developing infundibular stenosis. This generally becomes more marked with time. The over-riding aorta and the relative smallness of the left ventricle produce hypoxia and anaerobic respiration

INTRAVENOUS ANTI-ARRHYTHMIAL DRUGS

DRUG	DOSE	INDICATIONS	CAUTIONS
Aramine (Metaraminol)	0.3-2 mg/kg by IV drip in 500 cc D5W. Titrate.	PAT or PNT unresponsive to digitalis	Titrate to, do not exceed, maximum systolic BP of 140 to 160 mm Hg.
Digitalis Preparations	See section on Drug Doses.	Supraventricular arrhythmias: 1) PAT or PNT unresponsive to vagal stimulation. 2) Atrial flutter. 3) Atrial fibrillation.	Contraindicated in ventricular arrhythmias. May cause nausea, vomiting, varying degrees of heart block and arrhytmias.
Dilantin (Diphenylhydantion)	1 mg/kg dose. May repeat x 10 Maximum total dose = 500 mg over 4 hours.	1) Ventricular arrhythmias, especially ventricular tachycardia. 2) Digitalis-induced arrhythmias, especially Pat with block.	Excessive slowing of rate. (Discontinue drug until normal rate returns.)
Isuprel (Isoproteranol)	1-4 mg/liter; run in at 0.5-6.0 mcg per minute.	1) Complete heart block. 2) Severe bradycardia.	May cause pause palpitation, precordial pain, headache, tremor, or nausea.
Lidocaine (Xylocaine)	1 mg/kg slowly. Repeat PRN.	Ventricular arrhythmias.	May cause hypotension and CNS stimulation, including seizures, psychois and agitation.
Neosynephrine (Phenylephrine HCl)	10 mg (1 ml of 1% solution) in 100 cc D5W.	PAT or PNT unresponsive to digitalis.	Titrate to maximum systolic BP of 140-160 mm Hg. Bradycardia, atthythmias can occur.
Procaine Amide	2 mg/kg/dose in D5W, not faster than 0.5 mg/kg/ minute.	Ventricular tachycardia and ventricular flutter. Supraventricular arrhythmias unresponsive to digitalis.	Can also produce ventricular arrhythmias. May cause hypotension. Monitor EKG and BP q 1 min. While administering.
Propranalol	.025-.10 mg/kg IV by slow push. Maximum initial dose= 1 mg. Increase PRN.	Ventricular ectopic beats. Ventricular tachycardia. Digitalis-induced arrhythmias. Supraventricular tachycardia unresponsive to digoxin.	Hypotension and hypoglycemia may occur. Can produce bronchospasm; contraindicated in asthma.
Quinidine Sulfate	4 mg/kg/dose q2h for 4-5 doses.	Ventricular arrhythmias. Atrial flutter. Atrial fibrillation. May be used to prevent PAT in WPW syndrome.	Use in atrial arrhythmias only if patient is well digitalized. May cause widening of QRS complex, ventricular arrhythmias, tinnitis, nausea, vomiting and hypotension.

Chart 20.   Intravenous anti-arrythmial drugs.

which include the accumulation of pyruvic and lactic acid. This should be handled as an emergency and the acidemia should be corrected with bicarbonate, and shunt procedure performed, preferably an aortic-pulmonary window of approximately 3 mm in size. Once the shunting has provided a decrease in the hypoxemia, the acidemia corrects itself and hopefully the child will live for a long enough period of time until total correction becomes desirable. In any marked cyanosis, the correction of the acidemia is of paramount importance whether this be due to diaphragmatic hernia or any other causes of cyanosis.

INTERSEX

With the birth of an infant who has an intersex problem, a study of the sex chromatin is an integral part of the evaluation. Buccal smears from newborn females on the first day of life show a significant lower incidence of chromatin positive cells than is obtained from the normal adult female. This rapidly changes (*Pediatric Patient,* 1965).

The incidence of chromatin positive cells in the buccal smears in the newborn females in the first day of life varied from 6 to 37% (with a mean of 22%). By the fourth day of life, this had changed from 18 to 40% (with a mean of 29%).

Caution should be exercised, therefore, when interpreting the significance of a low chromatin count in the buccal smear before four days of age.

Suggested Reading

Pediatric Patient, 1965.

NEONATAL HYPOGLYCEMIA

Neonatal hypoglycemia may be very dangerous and is seen in approximately 30% of babies born of diabetic mothers. The theory behind the hypoglycemia is that during the latter part of gestation the mother runs a hyperglycemia and this stimulates the infant's pancreas to produce more insulin. Hypoglycemia, in the premature, is 20 mg% or below, whereas in the term baby it is 30 mg% or below. Optimally, these infants should be delivered between the 36th and 37th week of gestation to prevent too large an infant. Cord blood sugar should be done at about 3 hours of age and thereafter as frequently as necessary—especially if the infant is symptomatic. Of the 30% that develop hypoglycemia, 50% will have respiratory distress syndrome and this will account for the largest mortality. Respiratory distress syndrome is not only associated and aggravated by the hypoglycemia but there is also frequently an associated acidosis which potentiates the respiratory distress syndrome. Twenty-five per cent of the 30% with low blood sugar will have congenital malformations. Frequently, there is an associated increase in productivity of the adrenal cortex. The respiratory distress syndrome in the hypoglycemic infant usually commences in the first six hours of life. There is often hyperkalemia and hypocalcemia. An increased incidence of icterus is well known to occur in these infants.

The treatment should be aimed at moderate correction of hypoglycemia with 10% glucose, and if necessary, 25% or 50%, keeping in mind that if one gives the higher concentration of glucose it will potentiate further increase in insulin leading to a possible "vicious cycle." Correction of the hypoglycemia and relief of the respiratory distress syndrome is essential before any surgical correction can be undertaken to correct congenital malformations.

Suggested Reading

Cooke, Robt. E.: *The Biological Basis of Pediatric Practice,* McGraw Hill Book Co., New York.

CYSTO-UROGRAPHY

Cysto-urography is periodically very useful in the diagnosis of genitourinary disease. A good voiding urethrogram which avoids the hazards of retrograde studies is preferable and will suffice in the vast majority of diagnostic problems of a urological nature in pediatric surgical patients.

INDICATIONS FOR CYSTO-UROGRAPHY

1. Any child with clinical and/or laboratory findings of urinary tract infection.

A. First episode in male.
B. Second episode in female.
2. Other specific urinary symptoms, even without infection, enuresis, dysuria, hematuria, etc.
3. "Fever of unknown origin."
4. Other non-specific indications: Failure to thrive, megacolon, absent abdominal musculature, recurrent abdominal pain, other congenital anomalies.

PREPARATION

No special preparation is required for cystography alone. If cystography and intravenous pyelography are done simultaneously, intestinal cleansing and dehydration are carried out.

MATERIALS NEEDED

Catheter tray (disposable).
30 cc syringe (for opaque media) disposable.
5 cc syringe (for balloon catheter) disposable.
Catheters.
Normal saline.
Sterile basin.
Metal syringe adapter.
Hemostats.
Contrast media.

CONTRAST MEDIA

Sodium acetrizoate 30% (Cystokon Mallinckrodt) is used with the following dosage guide:

AGE GROUP	APPROXIMATE DOSE	DILUTION
Newborn – 3 months	40 – 60 cc	1:3 *
3 months – 2 years	60 – 90 cc	1:2
2 years – 5 years	90 – 120 cc	1:2
5 years – 7 years	120 – 150 cc	1:2
7 years – 15 years	150 – 200 cc	1:1

* One part Cystokon to three parts normal saline.

Cystokon has been found to produce excellent radio-opacity, is well tolerated, and is the least costly of the currently available cystographic media.

CYSTOGRAPHIC TECHNIQUE

1. A survey abdominal film taken (KUB).
2. All patients are then catheterized by the radiologist, using sterile technique. If a Foley type is used, the 3cc bag is inflated using sterile normal saline. Gentle traction is applied so that the balloon rests at the bladder neck.
3. Using a 30cc syringe, with an adapter tip, the bladder is slowly filled to capacity with contrast media. In the cooperative child, gravity alone may be used. In the younger or uncooperative patient, we introduce the opaque media via the syringe using gentle pressure.
4. Complete filling is determined in older children by their expression of fullness. In the younger child, the bladder dome can often be palpated. In addition, we have found that a dorsiflexed great toe (not unlike a positive Babinski reaction) is a reasonable end point for determining a full bladder.
5. An anterior-posterior abdominal radiograph is now exposed with the catheter in place. This corresponds to a "low pressure" study.
6. The child is then placed in the right lateral to right posterior oblique position and the catheter is removed.
7. The removal of the catheter will usually serve to initiate voiding. When the child will not, or cannot, void on command, gentle massage of the abdomen or the spraying of warm water on the genitalia will often produce the desired results.
8. Two or three films are exposed while the act of voiding is carried out. The lateral view is preferable for the demonstration of the bladder neck and urethra, but due to the thickness of the hips in older children, the oblique view is more commonly used.
9. An abdominal radiograph (KUB) is exposed as a "post voiding" study.

A number of investigators have reported good results using

cine, television tape, and spot film techniques. Because neither anesthesia nor premedication is required, many of the children can be examined as out-patients.

Suggested Reading

Altman, Donald H., *et al.:* Brochure, Variety Children's Hospital, Miami, Florida.

CARE OF THE TRACHEOSTOMY

Revolutionary to the care of the tracheostomy in infancy has been the introduction of silicone tracheostomy tubes. Prior to the introduction of these tubes by Dr. Louis Plzak of the Boston Children's Hospital, metal tubes were used which did not follow the contour of the infant's anatomy. The infant's trachea frequently bows forward during phases of respiration and the tubes were either too long or too short. The silicone tube however can be pared off with scissors, to proper length, to adapt together with the warmth of the body and its natural flexibility to follow the normal anatomy of the trachea in the infant. Of course one should avoid, if possible, a tracheostomy because of the dangers of not only keeping the trachea tube un-plugged but also the extreme hazard of "weaning" the child off the tracheostomy tube. The silicone tubes have an extra benefit bonus in that they remain clean with much less effort and they also come with a long arm on the exterior so that anesthesia administration is facilitated. The following is a suggested routine which has been used by the author satisfactorily in the care of tracheostomies:

MATERIALS

There should be a monel basin containing zephiran 1%. This is used to clean the endocath should the tracheostomy used have an endocath. (Silicone tubes do not require an endocath.)

Pipe cleaners used to clean the endocath. The endocath should be cleaned every 8 hrs. by someone knowledgable about the care of tracheostomies.

Sterile saline with a 2 cc syringe. This should be changed every 8 hrs. and the Zephiran changed every 8 hrs.

: endocath should be cleaned every 8 hrs. in 1% zephiran.
r. intervals, 3–4 drops of saline should be instilled into the
ıd the suction apparatus which has an adhesive marker
·rentially about the plastic aspiration catheter is placed
ɔuch a way as to preclude the person who is doing the suctioning going beyond the distal tip of the tracheostomy tube. Should
any bleeding occur, suctioning is then to be performed by an M.D.
only and one minim of adrenalin in ½ cc of saline is instilled into
the tracheostomy tube for hemostasis. All materials are kept under
sterile towels. The tracheostomy should be left in for as short a
period as possible. The longer the tracheostomy is in place the
more difficult it is to wean the infant from the tracheostomy.

When weaning the infant from the tracheostomy—a smaller tracheostomy tube is inserted to the point at which the child makes
a crying noise or is using his larynx and breathing without the
tube. A Q-tip cotton applicator is used to obtund the opening of
the smaller tracheostomy—this is placed ½ hour on and ½ hour off
and vital signs are closely monitored during this procedure. If
tolerated well for 24 hours, the tube is removed—preferably during morning hours so that the child can be closely observed and
vital signs are continued for an additional 24 hours.

HERNIAS, HYDROCELES AND UNDESCENDED TESTICLES

What could be new about these common-place problems? The
significance of a fluctuating hydrocele, which used to be treated
primarily by reassuring the parents, is now generally recognized
as associated with a communicating hernia above.

The presence of a short second toe or the apparent appearance
of a short second toe with a deep cleft between the great and
second toe in a consecutive series of 35 patients have all been associated with an indirect inguinal hernia. This is the first publica-
tion of this finding, and it should prove to be a highly accurate
sign for inguinal hernia.

The significant microscopic finding of advancing testicular
fibrosis after four years of age in the undescended testicle is a
strong point for correcting this condition between one and four
years of age, or certainly before school age. This finding has been

repeatedly confirmed by testicular biopsies. There are a number of advantages to early correction. Early correction is technically easier. The fibrosis is limited so that the size of the testicle is more normal and the cellular content healthier. The psychological stigma of being unlike other boys, which is more significant as the child gets older, is circumvented.

Suggested Reading

Owings, Richard S.: Recent Advances in Pediatric Surgery, *J M A Ga,* 52:3, March, 1963.

CONGENITAL HYPERTROPHIC PYLORIC STENOSIS

Pyloric stenosis is probably the most common abdominal surgical problem of infancy. Fifty years ago an infant with this condition faced an over-all mortality of 50 per cent. Today, in most institutions, the outlook for an infant with this condition is extremely bright in about 99 per cent of such cases. There is much speculation as to the possible etiology. Over-activity of the autonomic nervous system with resulting pylorospasm has been postulated as a precursor of pyloric stenosis, but there is little clinical evidence to support this contention. If that concept were valid, one might well expect an increased incidence of peptic ulceration in such individuals but this is not the case. A long term follow-up study by Ferguson and Jewett on a group of 56 patients operated at the Children's Hospital, Boston, failed to disclose an increased incidence of ulcer diasthesis. This study perhaps can be criticized somewhat in that the patients ranged from 24 to 32 years of age. Of the 56 patients, there was only one with a definite peptic ulcer and two additional patients who had symptoms suggestive of ulcer. The incidence of three in 56 compares favorably with previously reported figures of peptic ulcer in the population at large, but probably not for such a young age period. There may be some slight increase in the incidence of allergy in the background of patients with pyloric stenosis. In this particular series of 435 patients during a one year period of evaluation which roughly represents 75 patients, 15 had a history background of major allergy (asthma or eczema). An additional finding in this one-year period was that in eight patients there was one or more grandparent with diabetes, but no parents. Since diabetes tends to skip generations, this lead should be followed up and some determination made as to the subsequent incidence of diabetes in pyloric stenosis patients. The over-all mortality at the Boston Children's Hospital from 1953–59 in 435 patients was 0.69 per cent. Two of the three deaths were preventable—one due to an overwhelming staph pneumonia with septicemia—the other occurred in a depleted infant who vomited four days postoperatively and aspirated.

Suggested Reading

Owings, Richard S.: Recent Advances in Pediatric Surgery, *J M A Ga,* 52:3, March, 1963.

EXSTROPHY OF THE BLADDER AND CLOACA PROBLEMS

Exstrophy of the bladder has long been a controversial and difficult therapeutic problem. Several key anatomical observations have led to improvement in results including a higher percentage of urinary continence. Dr. Tague C. Chisholm of Minneapolis has emphasized certain points which have led to better long term results. Anatomical studies indicate that the sphincter is a splayed out ribbon which lies posterior to the exposed mucosa of the urethra and connects the diasthesis of the symphysis pubis. The nerve supply to the sphincter comes in right at the subperiosteal area. Former methods of repair were no doubt associated with severance of these nerve bundles. Also, it is important to remember that if the bladder can be turned in early, this larger bladder has less shrinkage and less redundant mucosa. Cracking the ilial wings bilaterally and rotating the symphysis pubis medially to re-connect these bones allows for three important results: (1) no dissection about the sphincter or its nerve supply is necessary (2) the sphincter can be re-approximated (3) the very important 90 degree angle between the bladder and the urethra can be developed. Dr. Chisholm reports on his experiences with 35 exstrophy patients and states that his results have steadily improved. Of his last 12 patients, all six of the females have good control, two of the boys have excellent control, two still dribble but are less than three years of age. One has a fistula at the vesico-urethral junction and one has a dehiscence. It is certainly encouraging that such good results are being obtained with this very difficult problem.

In regard to cloaca problems, again the recognition of the pathological anatomy holds the key to success. In this problem, in addition ot the associated imperforate anus, there is generally a bifid bladder separated by a strip of intestine which is the ileal-cecal valve region. It is tremendously important *not* to remove the unused tiny colon (once called the micro-colon). The first step in correction should be to free any associated omphalocele and the bifid bladders and then approximate the bladders in the midline, thereby creating an exstrophy. The ileal-cecal region should then be brought out as a cecostomy or colostomy and the micro-colon, if possible, brought through as an anal pull-through.

Suggested Reading

Rickman, P. P.: Vesico-Intestinal Fissure, *Arch Dis Child, 35*:97, 1960.
Chisholm, Tague C.: Exstrophy of the Urinary Bladder, *Am J Surg, 101*:649, 1961.

HIRSCHSPRUNG'S DISEASE

Hirschsprung's disease is characterized by the absence of the myenteric plexus in a segment of the large intestine. The lesion appears to be congenital, but its exact mechanism is unknown. Textbooks of embryology are remarkably reticent about the development of the plexus.

Laborious studies have been carried out which reveal a good deal about the function of the plexus. It should be noted that the gastro-intestinal wall contains two distinct nerve plexuses, one in the submucosa and the other between the two layers of the muscularis. The first, called the submucosal plexus or Meissner's plexus, consists almost entirely of non-myelinated post-ganglionic sympathetic fibers derived mainly from the superior mesenteric plexus. Meissner's plexus also contains a few ganglion cells that are part of the para-sympathetic system. Hence, some para-sympathetic preganglionic and post-ganglionic fibers must also be present in the plexus. The exact function of the plexus is not clear.

The other plexus, called the myenteric plexus or Auerbach's plexus, is somewhat better understood. It is situated mainly between the circular and the longitudinal muscle coats and is made up of nerve fibers and numerous ganglion cells. Most of the fibers are para-sympathetic in function. The preganglionic fibers are derived from the vagus nerve except in the distal part of the colon, where the plexus contains fibers derived from sacral autonomic structures. These fibers connect by synapses with the ganglion cells; the latter give off post-ganglionic fibers, most of which terminate on smooth muscle cells. These cells have a double innervation. They receive post-ganglionic sympathetic fibers directly from the cells of the pre-vertebral ganglia. These fibers of course comprise a part of Auerbach's plexus. Hence, the fibers of the plexus may be either sympathetic or para-sympathetic but the cells are all para-sympathetic in function. Whether or not the plexus contains afferent fibers is still a matter of controversy. However, there is good evidence that reflexes may originate in the gut wall and hence some sort of afferent mechanism must be present.

There is a general belief that para-sympathetic activity causes increased tone and motility of the gut muscles, and that sympathetic activity inhibits these functions. The absence of Auerbach ganglion cells in a segment of the colon explains the lack of peristaltic movement in this segment. It is interesting to note that the absence of Auerbach's plexus in the esophagus causes the dilated condition of the organ called achalasia.

Enterocolitis of Hirschsprung's Disease

Colostomy offers the best chance of success in treating the enterocolitis of Hirschsprung's disease in newborn infants. When enterocolitis appears for the first time after resection of the aganglionic segment, lateral sphincterotomy followed by repeated anal dilations by a member of the family is helpful. However, by preventing enterocolitis by colostomy as soon as Hirschsprung's disease is diagnosed in infancy, the mortality rate with megacolon can be reduced from 33% to 4%.

Pathogenesis

Enterocolitis is the chief cause of disability and death in Hirschsprung's disease and probably is related to partial mechanical intestinal obstruction by the aganglionic segment. Usually, symptoms of enterocolitis start in infancy but can occur at any age, either before or after abdomino-perineal resection.

Time of Onset

In the newborn infant, abdominal distention may be the first sign of enterocolitis, often beginning as early as the first or second day of life. Constipation and regurgitation of feedings, sometimes with bile staining, follow. After rectal dilation, all abnormal signs and symptoms may disappear, delaying further investigation. Explosive liquid diarrhea appears later, followed rapidly by hypovolemic shock. Unless intravenous treatment is given to restore circulating blood volume, the infant may die within twenty-four hours.

One cannot emphasize too greatly the importance of decompressing the bowel to allow for a small pull-through via a Duhamel or a Swenson precedure. It would be impossible to expect any satisfactory result from anastomosing a structure that is 4–5 inches in diameter with that of a 1 inch or less diameter.

Suggested Reading

Swenson, O., and Bill, A. H., Jr.: Resection of Rectum and Rectosigmoid with Preservation of the Sphincter for Benign Spastic Lesions Producing Megacolon, *Surgery, 24*:212, 1948.

Ehrenpreis, T.: Megacolon in the Newborn: A Clinical and Roentgenological Study with Special Regard to the Pathogenesis, *Acta Chir Scand, 94*:1, 1946.

Bill, Alexander H., Jr., and Chapman, Niles D.: The Enterocolitis of Hirschsprung's Disease, *Am J Surg: 103*:70, 1962.

INTUSSUSCEPTION

Should the treatment of intussusception be surgical or non-surgical? There should be no argument with the surgeon who wishes to attempt hydrostatic reduction of intussusception so long as the situation is of early duration. But once fever and "currant jelly" stools have occurred, both of which are late manifestations and connote jeopardized bowel and an impending deterioration of the child's general condition, such meddling should not be tolerated.

On the positive side for the use of hydrostatic pressure, the intussusception has been demonstrated repeatedly in children who have underlying gastrointestinal infections. Many of these cases spontaneously reduce. Properly performed, and provided there is no secondary evidence of bowel jeopardation, the low morbidity and mortality in Dr. Ravitch's series is quite impressive. This method of treatment has been used for many years but the most recent advocate in this country is Dr. Mark M. Ravitch. In his series of 67 patients reduced in this manner, there was only one death. Provided the barium is kept under the 3½ ft. level of height above the infant as recommended by Dr. Ravitch, the use of hydrostatic pressure has not been associated with perforation of bowel or reduction of gangrenous bowel. Two per cent of the children under 2 will have a specific lesion causing the intussusception, e.g., a polyp, Meckle's Diverticulum, or aberrant pancreatic tissue. These lesions will, of course, be missed if reduction occurs by barium enema. As Dr. Ravitch points out, controlled hydrostatic reduction of intussusception is a surgical procedure much as the reduction of a fracture by traction is a surgical procedure. The situation should be under direction of a surgeon who, in turn, should be ready to perform a laparotomy if it becomes necessary. The operating room should be alerted, and supportive measures initiated. We would conclude then that early in the course of illness when the child is in good general condition and is afebrile and has not passed "current jelly" stools, attempted reduction with hydrostatic pressure not to exceed 3½ ft. above the infant level is a useful procedure. Certainly, if one is able to demonstrate reflux of barium through the ileocecal valve, this is good evidence that there is no strangulation and that there has been a complete reduction. One misses the iteological process such as polyps, Meckle's Diverticulum, and aberrant pancreas but, on the other hand, these are not, in themselves, likely to be lethal problems. One also avoids operating on an infant who may well have enteritis or mesenteric adenitis which many feel are manifestations of a generalized illness.

It may be worthwhile to mention some of the symptoms aside from the colicky pain which generally occurs at from 3 to 5 minute intervals. The x-ray will generally show an empty right lower quadrant. In the abdominal examination, a mass will generally be felt just to the left of the midline in the abdomen. In the older infant, it may be necessary to sedate the child and for this 4 mg of nembutal/kg of body weight and 2 mg of demoral together may be given which will generally allow for a very satisfactory abdominal examination. It is imperative that the infant with an elevated temperature and pulse be adequately hydrated. One may even consider the introduction of oral neomycin if it is anticipated to take over six hours in preparation for surgery. A naso-gastric tube for decompression during the anesthesia is advisable. If the infant's condition is tenuous because of necrotic bowel, a Mickulicz exteriorization procedure as advocated by Dr. Ladd is the procedure of choice. This allows for a much shorter bowel resection at a subsequent time as well as for a clean anastomosis. A primary aseptic anastomosis may also be performed if the child's condition is adequate and time permits. The presence of Meckle's Diverticulum which is the beginning of the intussusception with its subsequent edema should be handled much as a diseased appendix.

Suggested Reading

Ravitch, M.: Non-operative Treatment of Intussusception; Hydrostatic Pressure Reduction by Barium Enema, *Surg Clin N Am: 36*:1495, 1956.

IMPERFORATE ANUS

In patients with imperforate anus Erhenpries noted that there is a decrease in the ganglion cells in the lower extent of the imperforate bowel and the farther one goes cephalad the more likely one is to run into a normal number of ganglion cells. These patients appear to have a relative Hirschsprung's and one should be aware of this when bringing down the bowel to bring down bowel that has an adequate number of ganglion cells. Much has been written about the importance of the pubo-rectalis sling which is very important for continence. The bowel must be brought through this sling. Should this not be possible, one may do a Kottmier procedure which consists of taking down the posterior lateral attachment of the pelvic diaphragm and making a large anteriorly based pubo-rectalis sling. This muscle band is approximated behind the rectum. Imperforate anus and Hirschsprung's disease are probably inter-related and one should have a thorough knowledge of the local anatomy before attempting surgical correction.

Suggested Reading

Owings, Richard S.: Recent Advances in Pediatric Surgery, *J M A Ga: 52*:3, March 1963.

OXYGEN IN THE NEWBORN

The catastrophic effects of oxygen therapy for the premature as a cause of retrolental fibroplasia poses the sobering question of how much oxygen should be given to the respiratory-distressed infant. The question of how much oxygen is safe remains unanswered. Certainly the cyanotic infant or a premature having intermittent apnea needs oxygen. Surgeons frequently use high oxygen content to decrease post-operative distention associated with abdominal surgery. The following points can be made:

(1) Infants of more than 35 weeks gestation can be placed in oxygen without known risks.

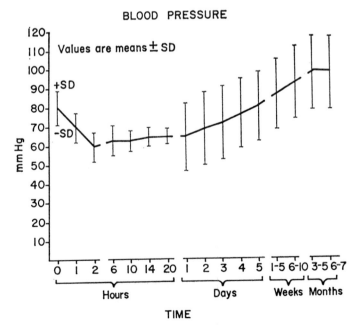

Chart 21. Blood pressure variations with age of infant.

(2) The presence of cyanosis is the best possible justification for use of oxygen but unnecessary risks should be avoided.

(3) Periodically the oxygen should be turned off and the infant watched carefully to see whether the cyanosis returns.

(4) 40% oxygen in nitrogen in constant use may be justified in the apneic immature infant but constant nursing care and frequent use of physical stimuli to ward off apenea may be a great deal safer.

Suggested Reading

Avery, M. E., *et al.: J Appl Physiol, 18*:895, 1963.

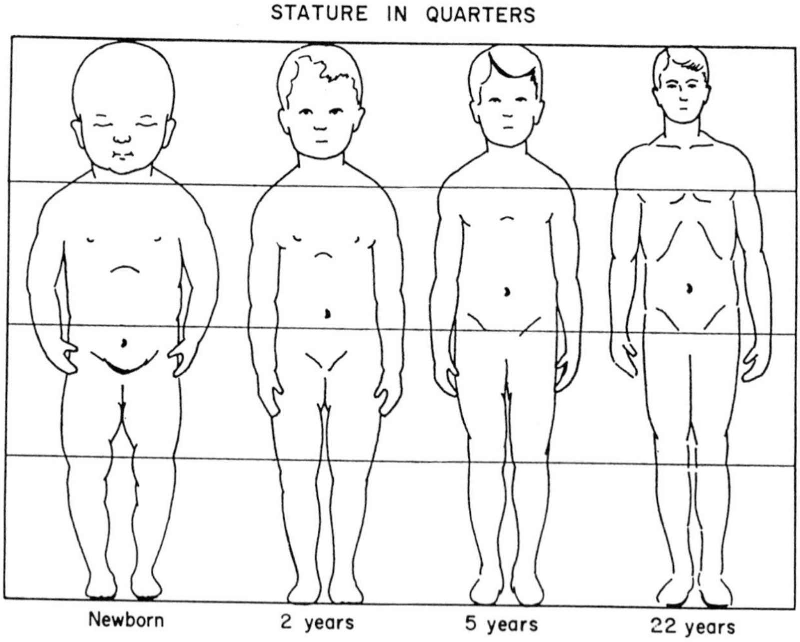

STATURE IN QUARTERS

Newborn   2 years   5 years   22 years

Chart 22.   Crown: Rump maturation with age.

MECHANISM OF TUMOR ANGIOGENESIS:

Therapeutic Implications

Dr. Judah Folkman, of the Children's Hospital Medical Center, Boston, Massachusetts, has isolated a factor from solid tumors

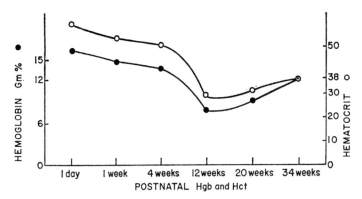

Chart 23. Postnatal hemoglobin and hematocrit.

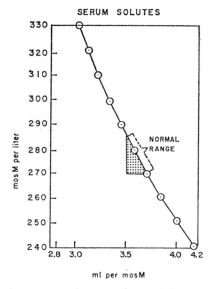

Chart 24. *Osmolarity range of human plasma.* The range of the osmolarity of the serum is between rather narrow limits is illustrated in this chart.

which is mitogenic to capillary endothelial cells and results in rapid neovascularization. Tumor-angiogenesis-factor (T.A.F.) has been found in mouse and rat tumors and in hepatoblastoma, neuroblastoma, rhabdomyosarcoma, and Wilm's tumors from nine patients. It is not present in normal tissues except for placenta. Its important components are RNA and protein. Its molecular weight is approximately 100,000. It is inactivated by ribonuclease and at 56° C.

Parallel experiments with tumor implants in more than 100 isolated perfused organs demonstrate that blockade of angiogenesis stops expansion of most tumors at a diameter of 2–3 mm.

From these two lines of investigation, Dr. Folkman has developed a new working hypothesis for the life cycle of solid malignancy. A tumor colony arising from a single cell or from a clump of cells within a metastasis expands until it exceeds the limits of simple *diffusion* of nutrients; growth pauses. The tumor releases a humoral signal (T.A.F.) which stimulates neighboring capillaries to form new sprouts. When these reach the tumor, nutrients are supplied by *perfusion* and exponential growth begins anew.

Dr. Folkman suggests that the most vulnerable period in the life of a solid tumor may be the brief interval before vascularization. If this is true, "anti-angiogenesis" therapy, perhaps by immunization against T.A.F., should provide a powerful adjunct to cancer surgery. Tiny recurrent tumors, held dormant in the unvascularized state may prove to be harmless, or at least more susceptible to chemotherapy and radiotherapy.

Suggested Reading

Folkman, Judah: Original Paper Presented Second Annual Meeting, *Am. Ped. Surg. Assoc.,* 1971.

Chapter 24

LIFE LINE: TOTAL PARENTERAL NUTRITION IN INFANTS WITH CATASTROPHIC GASTROINTESTINAL ANOMALIES

I have used total parenteral maintenance of numerous puppies and a number of human patients with good success. I have corresponded with Dr. Stanley J. Dudrick of the University of Pennsylvania who is one of the pioneers in this work. The following is a summary of some of the work that has led to this great advance in maintaining these very seriously ill infants.

Intensive nutritional support is essential for survival and surgical rehabilitation of newborn infants with gastronintestinal anomalies. Oral feedings can usually be established after correction of a single congenital defect. At times, a feeding tube or gastrostomy may be required to provide nutrients to poor risk infants. However, all too often, internal feeding is impossible and parenteral support inadequate, so that babies with multiple or complex lesions of the gastrointestinal tract die from the complications of starvation.

The laboratory demonstration that normal growth and development can be achieved by supplying basic nutrients exclusively by the intravenous route prompted use of the technique in surgical patients. More than 200 adults with chronic complicated gastrointestinal disease have been supported exclusively by the intravenous route with 2400–5000 calories per day for 10 to 200 days. Weight gain was observed in all patients associated with wound healing, fistula closure, positive nitrogen balance, and increased strength and activity.

Preliminary data on the first infant to be nourished by this intravenous feeding technique demonstrated normal growth, development, and metabolism despite near total absence of the small bowel and gastrointestinal dysfunction. This is the first infant in whom total parenteral nutrition was used in conjunction with surgical treatment of catastrophic gastrointestinal anomalies.

Chart 25.   PEDIATRIC HYPERALIMENTATION SOLUTION PREPARATION

Unit Preparation of Base Solution	
	(20 gm hydrolysates
400 ml 5% dextrose in 5% fibrin hydrolysate	160 kcal(20 gm dextrose
250 ml 50% dextrose	500 kcal
650 ml	660 kcal
Addition to Each Unit of Base Solution	
Sodium Chloride	10 ml
(2 mEq/ml)	
Potassium phosphate, monobasic	13 ml
(2 mEq/ml)	
Calcium gluconate 10%	44 ml
(0.45 mEq/ml)	
Magnesium sulfate 50%	1.2 ml
(8 mEq/ml)	
Added to solution daily or weekly or given	1 ml
intramuscularly	
Added to solution daily or given as 10 ml/kg	1 ml
plasma twice weekly	
	75 ml
Base solution	650 ml	
Additives	75 ml	
Final solution	725 ml	(Given at rate of 145 ml/kg/day = 130 kcal/kg/day)

Total parenteral nutrition can be placed into either the inferior or superior vena cava via a silicone I.V. tube. This can be introduced by way of a large thin wall needle in the subclavian and threading the silicone tube into the superior vena cava or one can, after meticulously cleansing the inguinal area, place a cannula through the saphenous bulb into the inferior vena cava. Both wound areas have to be kept carefully clean either by an occlusive dressing or with the use of antibiotic ointment at frequent intervals. Silicone catheters thus introduced can be used for months without difficulty. This author has used "life-line" tubes upwards to two months in severe burns without any evidence of phlebitis or other difficulties.

Total parenteral nutrition in 18 infants with multiple or complex anomalies allowed growth, development, increased activity, wound healing, and survival despite prolonged dysfunction of the intestinal tract and repeated operative procedures. Successful surgical rehabilitation of infants with catastrophic gastrointestinal anomalies is possible with total intravenous feedings and well planned operative treatment.

Suggested Reading

Dudrick, Stanley J., *et al.:* New Horizons for Intravenous Feeding, *JAMA, 215*:6, Feb. 8, 1971.

Dudrick, Stanley J., *et al.:* Total Parenteral Nutrition in Infants with Catastrophic Gastrointestinal Anomalies, *J Ped Surg: 1*:2, Apr., 1969.

Report of Committee on Nutrition, American Academy of Pediatrics, *Pediatrics, 46*:4, July 1972.

Committee on Nutrition: Parenteral Feeding—A Note of Caution. *Pediatrics, 49*:5, May, 1972.

INDEX

A

Acheson, R. M.; Paul, R. M. and
    Tomlinson, R.V., 78
Acidosis, and alkalosis, metabolic,
    17
ACTH, 47–48
Acidemia, 118
Adhesions, prevention of, 34
Adrenal insufficiency, 23
Ahmed, I., 32
Alderhey Clinic, 36
Alkali, replacing, 29
Alkalosis, and acidosis, 17
Altman, Donald H. *et al.,* 122
Amino acid, extracted by liver, 28
Ampicillin, 58
Analgesia, 50
Anesthesia,
    administration of, 53
    endotracheal intubation and ven-
        tilation, 51
    general, 52–55
    goals of, 50–51
    of premature infant, problems in,
        50
Anderson, C. M., and Freeman, M.,
    105
Angiogenesis, mechanism of tumor,
    132
Anti-arrythmial drugs, Intravenous,
    117
Antibiotics, 56–61
    aminoglycosides, 56
    Ampicillin, 58
    Bacitracin, 60
    bactericidal, 56
    bacteriostatic, 56
    Carbenicillin, 59

cyclic polypeptides, 56
Erythromycin, 59
Garamycin, 59
Gentamicin, 59
Geopen, 59
in uremia, 63
Kanomycin, 58
Kantrex, 58
Keflin, 60
Lincomycin, 59
Neomycin, 60
neonate's response to, 56–61
Novabiocin, 60
Oxytetracycline, 60
penicillin, 57
Polyene, 56
Polymyxin, 60
streptomycin, 58
sulfonamides, 58
Terramycin, 60
tetracyclines, 58
Anti-fungal agents, 56
Anus, imperforate, 130
Apnea, course of, 42
Armstrong, M. D.; McMillan, A.,
    and Shaw, K. N. F., 78
Asphyxiation, 64–65
Atresia, esophageal, 95
Avery, M. E., *et al.,* 132
Avery, M. E., 99
Ayre's T-piece, 53

B

Barnett, H. L., 18, 27, 61, 105
Bellious, F.; Beaz, J., and Shumack-
    er, H. E., 89, 92

139

Bigler, J. A., and McQuiston, W. O., 45
Bill, Alexander, 75, 78, 80
Bill, A. H., Jr., 128
Biochemical and physiological Reactions of the Neonate to Surgery, 36–41
  fluids, 39
  nitrogen, 40
  potassium balance, 38
  temperature, 39
Bladder, exstrophy of and cloaca problems, 125
Blood pressure, 131
Blood replacement, 53, 113
Bockman, Leonard, 112
Body fluids, 19
Body Metabolism, 28–30
  during starvation, 28–29
  during trauma, 29–30
Body surface in relation to weight, 23
Body warmth in care of premature infant, 51
Boston Children's Hospital, X
Brij, M. L. K., et al., 35
Browne, Sir Denis, VII
BUN, 16, 17, 39
Burns, 64–69
  estimating body surface, 64
  complications, 64
  treatment of, 65–68
Burroughs, Milton, X

C

Caldwell, Velma, X
Cancer, in Childhood, 69–94
  bone tumors, 87
  Hodgkin's disease, 85
  lipoblastoma, 89
  lymphohemangioma, 92
  lymphosarcoma, 86
  neuroblastoma, 69–80
    diagnosis of, 72
    recent thoughts concerning, 78
    therapy of, 74
  rhabdomyosarcoma, 83
  retinoblastoma, 81
  Wilm's tumor, 81

Carbenicillin (Geopen), 59
Carbohydrates, fats and protein, 28
Carbon dioxide elimination, proper, 53
Cardiac arrest, 33–34
Cardiac reserve, 42–43
Chapman, Niles D., 128
Charts
  Therapy of infections, 61–63
  Pediatric procedures, 114
Chemical equivalents and chemical pressures, 23
Children's hospitals, X
Children's medical centers, need for, 6
Chisholm, Tague C., 126
Chloride, 18
Chloromycetin, 56
Chlorpromazine, 46
Christensen, H. N., et al., 41
Christy, N. P.; Knight, M.; Langston, D., and Jailer, J. W., 49
Clatworthy, H. W., Jr., 95
Cloaca Problems and exstrophy of the bladder, 125
Collin's rule, 82
Committee on Nutrition, report of, 137
Complications and their prevention, 31–35
  adhesions, prevention of, 34
  heavy drapes, 35
  hypernatremia, 31
  hyperthermia, 32
  hypothermia, 33
Congenital hypertrophic pyloric stenosis, 124
Constituents, plasma comparison, 21
Cooke, Robert E., 30, 119
Corticosteroid, excretion, 38, 46
Cyanosis, 116, 118
Cyanotic congenital heart disease, 116
Cyclic polypeptides, 56
cyclophosphamide, 77
cyclopropane and ether, 52, 46
Cystographic technique, 121
Cystokon, 120
Cysto-urography, 119–120

D

Dactinomycin, 76, 77
Darrow-Yennet concept, 17
Darrow's solution, 40
DeBoer, Arthur, 45
Decamethonium, 53
De-cannulating a child, 55
Dehydration, hypernatremia, 31
Denis, J., *et al.,* 100
Depletion
  salt, 19
  water, 19
Dexamethasone, 34–35
Diagnosis, X
  of neuroblastoma, 72
  and therapy of tumor, 74
Diaphragmatic hernia, VIII, 100
  and omphalocele, similarity be-
    tween, 98
Diet, low-salt, 23
Dislocation of hip, VIII
DNA, 115
Drapes
  heavy in infant, 35, 42
  complications in surgery, 35
Dudrick, Stanley J., 135, 137
D-tuborcurarine, use of in infants,
  53
Duodenal ulcers, 108

E

Edwards, K. M.; Jepson, R. P., and
  Reese, M. W., 49
Ehrenpreis, T., 128
Eik-Nes, K., 49
Electrolytes: 13–27
  and fluids, 19–27
  and fluid replacement in the op-
    erative newborn, 13–18
  water, sodium and potassium re-
    quirements, 15
Emery, J. L., 38, 41
Endocrine, response to surgery, 43
Endotracheal intubation and venti-
  lation, 51, 52
Engstron respirator, 54
Enterocolitis of Hirschsprung's dis-
  ease, 127–128

Equivalents, chemical and pressures,
  23
Eraklis, *et al.,* 101
Erythromycin and Lincomycin, 59
Esophageal
  fistulas, 94
  lye ingestion, 96
  varices, 105
Essentials of pediatric surgery, VII
Ether, 46, 52
Ewings sarcoma, 88
Exstrophy of the bladder and cloaca
  problems, 125, 126

F

Fats, carbohydrates and protein, 28
Finberg, L., 32
Fisher, John H., 110
Fistulas, tracheo-esophageal, 94
Fluid
  and electrolyte replacement in op-
    erative newborn, 13–18
  and electrolyte management, prin-
    ciples in, 16
  and electrolytes, 19, 24
  body consist of, 19
  compartments in infant and ad-
    ults, 21
  intravenous, 16, 26
  oral volume intake, 13
  rough guide to replacement, 39
Fluothane, 52
Folkman, Judah, 75, 132, 134
Franksson, C.; Gamzell, C. A., and
  vonEuler, U. S., 49
Franksson, C. *et al.,* 46
Freeman, M., 105

G

Gainza, E., 49
Garamycin, 64, 67
Gardner, L. I., 78
Gastrointestinal anomalies, 135
Gellis, S. S., and Holt, L. E., Jr., 97
Gellis, S. S., and Kagan, B. M., 61
Gemzell, C. A., 49
General anesthesia, 52

Gentamicin, 59
Geopen, 59
G. I. bleeding associated with esoph-
    ageal varices, 105
Glucose concentration, 28
Goals of anesthesia, 50
Gray Syndrome, 56
Gross, Robert, 111
Gross, R. E., 103
Growth chart—premature, 14
Guide
    preoperative medication, 51
    therapy for infection, 61
Guillemin, R.; Rosenberg, B., 48, 49

H

Hancock, John, Life Insurance, 3
Hand, A. M., and Leininger, C. R.,
    45
Handling of Newborn, 11
Harvard Medical School, X
Heavy drapes in infants, 35
Helmreich, M. L., 47, 49
Hernia
    diaphragmatic, 100
    hydroceles and undescended testi-
        cles, 123
Hill, Fontain S., 27
Hirschsprung's disease, X, 126
    enterocolitis of, 127–128
Hodgkin's disease, 85
Holinger, P. H., *et al.*, 97
Holt, L. E., Jr., 97
Hormonal fluctuation in pediatric
    surgery, 46–49
Hospital for Sick Children, The, IX
Hume, D. M., and Nelson, D. H.,
    49
Humidification, 54
HVA, 75–76
Hydroceles, undescended testicles
    and hernias, 123
Hydroxycorticosteroids, 46
Hypernatremia, dehydration, 31
Hyperthermia
    in shock, 32, 33, 43
    results of, 33
Hypnosis, 50

Hypoglycemia, 46
    neonatal, 118
Hypokalemia, 40
Hypothermia
    cardiac arrest and shock, 33–34
    results of, 33
Hypoxia, 42

I

Ileus, 13
    meconium, 104
Imperforate anus, 130
Incidence of Pediatric Surgery, 3–5
Infant, problems in anesthetizing a
    premature, 50
Infection
    in burns, 64
    guide to therapy, 61
Ingestion, lye, 96
Insensible water loss, 39
Insulin, 29
Intake-output Record, 25
Intersex, 118
Intestinal obstruction, 13
Intra-uterine surgery, 114
Intravenous: anti-arrythmial drugs,
    117
    fluids, 16, 26
    infusion, 40, 67
Intubation, ventilation endotrache-
    al, 51
Intussusception, 128, 129, 130

J

Jailer, J. W., 49
James, David H., Jr., 69, 77, 89
Jeffner and Kaplan, 4
Jenkins, D., 49
Jepson, R. P., 49
Jones, P. G., 102

K

Kagan, B. M., 61
Kanamycin, 58
Kaplan, 4

Kaser, Von H.; Schweisguth, D.; Sellio, K., and Spengler, G. A., 78

Kauffman, S. L., and Stout, A. P., 92

Keflin, 60

Keterosteroid excretion, 38

Kieswetter, W. B., 103

Kilograms, square meter of body surface to body weight, 23

Knight, M., 49

Koop, C. Everett, 76, 96, 112

Koop and Owings, *et al.*, 92

L

LaBrosse, Elwood H., 76

Ladd, Wm. E., VIII, IX

Langston, D., 49

Laparotomy, 106

Lee, C. Marshall, 3, 5

Leininger, C. R., 45

Leubner, H., 105

Life Line: Total Parenteral Nutrition in Infants with Catastrophic Gastrointestinal Anomalies, 135

Lincomycin and Erythromycin, 59

Lipoblastoma, 89

Local anesthesia for abdominal surgery, 12, 52

Long, C. N. H., 49

Longino, Luther, 94

Loss, insensible water, 15

Low salt diet, 23

Lungs, response to surgical stress, 42

Lye ingestion, 96

Lymphocytes, 78, 79

Lymphosarcoma, 86

M

Malignant tumors of children, 69

McCance, R. A., 41, 38

McCance, R. A., and Young, W. F., 45

McKay, R. J., 105

McMillen, A., 78

McQuiston, W. O., and Bigler, J. A., 43, 45

Mechanism of tumor angiogenesis, 132

Mecker, I. A., 68

Meconium ileus, 104, 106

Medical College of Georgia, X, 3

Metabolic
acidosis, 17
alkalosis, 17
homeostasis, 18, 24, 20, 27
surgical care, 27

Metabolism during starvation and trauma, 28

Metabolite of norepinephrine, 78

Metcoff, J., *et al.*, 68

Milliequivalents, 17
of chloride, 18
to convert milligrams % to, 25
milliosmol, 26

Mingeon, Claude J., 49

Miscellaneous
subjects, 111
tumors, 89

Molar solution, 25

Monitor without handling, 112

Moore, Francis D., 27

Moore, T. C., *et al.*, 35

Morgan, Allen, 80

Mucoviscidosis, 104, 105

Murphy, D. R., *et al.*, 101

Muscular relaxation, 50

N

Need for more regional total care children's medical centers, 6

Nelson, D. H., 49

Nelson, W. E., Vaughan, V. C., and McKay, R. J., 105

Neomycin and Polymyxin, 60

Neonatal hypoglycemia, 118

Neonate, the biochemical and physiological reactions to surgery, 36

Neonates response to antibiotic, uses and abuses, 56

Neostigmine—used to reverse action of D-tubocurarine, 53

Nephroblastoma—Wilm's tumor, 81

Nitrous oxide, 52, 53

Neuroblastoma, 69
diagnosis of, 72, 74

some recent thoughts concerning, 78
Newborn
    handling of, 11
    operative, fluid and electrolyte replacement, 13
    oxygen in the, 131
    surgery of, 11
    temperature, 37
Nitrogen—excretion during postoperative period, 38
No Trendelenberg for long periods in newborn, 112
Norepinephrine—metabolite, 78
Novabiocin, 60
Nutrition in infants with catastrophic gastrointestinal anomalies, 135

O

Obstruction, intestinal, 13
Obtundation of reflex, 51
Omphalocele, 102
Omphalocele, similarity between patient with diaphragmatic hernia and, 98
Operative newborn, fluid and electrolyte replacement, 13
Oral fluid volume intake, 13
Osmolarity range of human plasma, 133
Osteogenic sarcoma, 87
Output-intake record, 25
Owings, Helen, X
Owings and Koop, *et al.*, 92
Owings, Richard S., 10, 89, 124, 125, 131
Owings, Richard S., and Radakovich, Michael, 89
Oxygen
    adequate, 11
    in the newborn, 131
Oxytetracycline (terramycin), 60

P

Paradox, sodium and retention, 23
Parenteral nutrition, 137

Pathogenesis, 127
Paul, R. M., 78
Pediatric hyperalimentation solution preparation, 136
Pediatric medicine, 4
Pediatric Surgery
    definition of, IX
    hormonal fluctuation in, 46
    incidence of, 3–5
    maxims, 111
Penicillin, 57
Pentothal, 46
Peptic ulcer, 108
Phenolic acids, 78
Physician
    to population ratio, 7–8
    time requirements, 9
Pickel, S., 32
Plasma
    constituents, 21
    neonatal, 19
Polk, H. C., and Stone, H. H., 68
Polymyxin, 60
Post-operative
    adhesions, 34–35
        causes, 34
        prevention, 34–35
    pyloric position, 114
    sodium and chloride retention, 37
    water retention, 37
    weight loss, 37
Potassium
    balance, 36–38, 40
    carbonate, 72
    plasma concentration in newborn, 15
    requirements, 15–18
    shift, absence of, 37
    water and sodium requirements, 15
Potts, Willis, V
Premature
    growth chart, 14
    problems in anesthetizing, 50
Pre-operative orientation of patient, 5
Pressures, chemical and equivalents, 23
Promethazine, 34–35
Protein, carbohydrates and fats, 28

Pyloric position, post-operative, 114
Pyloric Stenosis, congenital hyper-
    trophic, 124
Pyloroplasty, Hinecke-Mickulicz, 96

R

Radakovich, Michael, 89
Radiation therapy, 77, 85
Raffensperger, John G., *et al.,* 110
Rastick, M. M., *et al.,* 101
Ravitch, M. M., 129, 130
Reaction of neonate to surgery, 36–
    41
    biochemical, 37–41
    physiological, 36–37
    shock, 113
Record, intake-output, 25
Rectal prolapse, 104
Reese, M. W., *et al.,* 46, 49
Regional total care children medi-
    cal centers, 6
Renal
    shut-down with potassium intoxi-
        cation, 64–65
    system, 43
Replacement, blood, 53
    fluid and electrolyte, 13
Replogle, Robert L., 35
Reserpine, 46
Respiratory
    distress syndrome, 111
    reserve of infants, 54
Response
    to antibiotics, uses and abuses, 56
    to surgical stress, 42–45
        cardiac reserve, 42–43
        endocrine system, 43
        lung action, 42
        renal system, 43
Retention, sodium, 23
Retinoblastoma, 81
Rhabdomyosarcoma, 83
Rickman, P. P., 36, 41
Rosenberg, B., 49
Rule, Collin's, 82
Rule of Seven's, in burns, 64, 113
Rule of Thirteen, burns in infants,
    113

S

Salt
    depletion, 19
    urinary, 23
Salzer method, in lye ingestion, 97
Samuels, L. T., 49
Sandberg, A. A., *et al.,* 20
Sarcoma
    Ewings, 88
    osteogenic, 87
Sayers, G., 49
Schumacker, H. E., 92
Schweisguth, O., 78
Seller, K., 78
Sevens, Rule of, in burns, 64
SGOT and SGPT, 59
Shaw, K.N.F., 78
Shirkey, H. C., 61
Shock
    acute fluid loss, 65
    hyperthermia, 32
    unremitting, 64
Shwackman, H., and Leubner, H.,
    105
Silverman, Wm. A., 34
Smith, C. A., 41
Smith, J. W., 61
Smith, Robert M., 50, 51, 55
Sodium
    nitrate solution, 72
    paradox, 23
    pentobarbital, 46
    replacement, inadequate, 15
    requirements, 15–17
    water, and potassium, 15
Spengler, G. A., 78
Square meter of body surface, 23
Stage procedures, 112
Starvation and trauma, metabolism
    during, 28
Statland, Harry, 24, 27
Stone, H. H., 68
Stooner, H. B., Whiteley, H. J., and
    Emory, J., 41
Stout, A. P., 92
Stress, prevention of surgical, 43–45
Sulfamyalon, 64, 67
Sulfonamides, 58
Surgery
    biochemical and physiological re-

actions of neonate, 36
intra-uterine, 114
of the newborn, 11–12
Surgical
loss of children and why, 114
maxims, 111
patients, percent of, 3
stress, 42
Suxamethonium, 53
Swan, H., 49
Swenson, O., and Bill, A. H., Jr., 128
Syndrome, respiratory distress, 111

T

Talbott, Nathan B., 18, 23, 24, 27
Temperature, in newborn, 39
Terramycin, 60
Tetracyclines, 58
Tetralogy of Fallot, 117
Therapy
of infections, guide to, 61
tumor, 74
Thomas, J. P., Owen, *et al.*, 111
Thomasson, B. H., 49
Tomlinson, R. V., 78
Tracheo-esophageal fistulas, 94
Tracheostomy, 54
care of, 122
Transposition of the great vessels, 117
Trauma, 29
metabolism during, 28
Tumor
angiogenesis, mechanism of, 132
diagnosis and therapy, 74
of the bone, 87
malignant in children, 69
miscellaneous, 89
Tyler, F. H., 49

U

Ulcer, peptic, 108
Undescended testicles, hernias and hydroceles, 123
University Hospital, 3
of Pennsylvania, X
of Rochester, X
Uremia, antibiotics in, 63

V

Van Meurs, V. P., 92
Vaughn, C. C., 101
Vaughan, V. C., 105
Ventilator, 54
Ventilation, endotracheal intubation and, 51
Ventricular septal defect, 117
Vesico-intestinal fissure, 126
Viikari, S. J., and Thomasson, B. H., 49
Vincrystine sulfate, 77
Virtue, R. W.; Helmreich, M. L., and Gainza, E., 49
VMA, 75–76
Von Euler, U. S., 49
Von Studnitz, W., 78
Voorhess, M. L., and Gardner, L. I., 78

W

Wall, P. E., 78
Ward, Sir Lancelot Barrington, IX, 111
Water
abnormal loss of, 15
depletion, 19
insensible loss, 15
retention, post-operative, 37
sodium and potassium requirements, 15
Weight
in relation to body surface, 23–24
loss, post-operative, 37
White, Harvey, 107
Whiteley, H. J., 41
Wilkinson, A. W., 55, 81
Wilm's tumor (nephroblastoma), 81
Wolfson, S. A., *et al.*, 101

Y

Yennet-Darrow concept, 17
Young, W. F., 45

Z

Zollinger, R. M., 110